D0673376

# CHRIS RYAN'S
# SAS
# FITNESS
# BOOK

# CHRIS RYAN'S
# SAS
# FITNESS
# BOOK

Century

Published by Century in 2004

7 9 10 8 6

Copyright © Chris Ryan 2000
Foreword copyright © Chris Ryan 2004

Chris Ryan has asserted his right under the Copyright, Designs and
Patents Act, 1988, to be identified as the author of this work

This book is sold subject to the condition that it shall not, by way of
trade or otherwise, be lent, resold, hired out, or otherwise circulated
without the publisher's prior consent in any form of binding or cover
other than that in which it is published and without a similar condition
including this condition being imposed on the subsequent purchaser

First published in the United Kingdom in 2000 by Century
The Random House Group Limited
20 Vauxhall Bridge Road, London SW1V 2SA

www.randomhouse.co.uk

Addresses for companies within The Random House Group Limited
can be found at: www.randomhouse.co.uk/offices.htm

The Random House Group Limited Reg. No. 954009

A CIP catalogue record for this book is available
from the British Library

The Random House Group Limited supports The Forest
Stewardship Council (FSC), the leading international forest
certification organisation. All our titles that are printed on
Greenpeace approved FSC certified paper carry the FSC logo.
Our paper procurement policy can be found at:
www.randomhouse.co.uk/environment

ISBN 9781844138098

Typeset in Rotis Serif and Rotis Sans Serif

Design & make up by Roger Walker

Printed and bound in Great Britain by
Scotprint

*To Janet and Sarah*
(keep going girls)

## ACKNOWLEDGEMENTS

I would like to thank the following:

My editor, Anna Cherrett, and the rest of the team at Random House; Paul Rooney for his help in the beginning, also Dean and Caroline for pushing me so hard in the last few months of this project; and, last but not least, my agent, Barbara Levy.

The purpose of this book is to give the reader general information on the subjects of fitness training and weight lifting. Although the guidelines and advice have been sourced from or reviewed by sources believed to be reliable some aspects of the book may not be suited to every reader and can depend on the level of fitness and health the reader brings to the book as well as age and other factors. Readers are strongly advised to consult with their doctor and seek the guidance of professional fitness experts before beginning any of the fitness programmes or activities contained within.

# Contents

# Foreword to new edition

In the four years since this book was first published, perceptions about fitness and body weight have seen a few changes. For example, it's now accepted that our genes have an enormous influence on how much we eat. In other words we're programmed to eat the way we do.

That's not a problem if you have to go foraging for food. It's not even that big a deal when you have to buy the ingredients raw and then go home to cook them. But it does seem to be an issue now that every corner shop has stacks of high fat snacks, and the ready-meals and takeaways we're addicted to as a nation are fairly dripping with the stuff.

The problem seems to be that we can't ignore these invitations to gorge because hundred of thousands of years of evolution have programmed us to store up fat whenever and wherever we can.

But that's not all.

As junk food spreads everywhere, we're taking less and less exercise. Labour saving devices have all but eliminated hard chores in the home and outside the home we drive everywhere. School sports have suffered enormously since local councils starting selling off playing fields. Because kids are discouraged from mucking around outside in their spare time, they're more likely to be found sitting on their backsides in front of a video game than kicking a football.

It's a pincer movement with only one result: an epidemic of obesity.

It's my belief that getting fit is by far the best way of losing weight.

Let's go back to basics. The only way you're going to lose weight is by burning up more calories than you're taking in. There are only two ways of doing this: eating less and exercising more. While I watch what I eat, the reason I've written Chris Ryan's Exercise Book and not Chris Ryan's Diet Book is simple: I believe that all the odds are stacked against a diet helping you lose weight in the long term.

In fact, I'd go as far as to say that weight-loss diets offer the worst of all worlds.

For a start, they're based on giving up things you like, so right from the off you're working against the grain *and* feeling lousy, likely as not. Secondly, sticking to a diet is a demanding, full time job. You're surrounded by temptation every minute of every day. Thirdly, when you do fall off the wagon – and everyone does – you're inclined to put on even *more* weight than before. Your body has slowed its metabolism right down in order to try and hang on to its store of fat. Again, that's what it's been programmed to do by evolution.

If diet's the lose-lose option, fitness offers a win-win solution. Far from giving anything up, you're gaining all the way along the line: picking up new skills, boosting your self-esteem, doing wonders for your health and improving your appearance. What's more, you're in control. If you want a blow-out or an evening down the pub, go ahead and enjoy it. It's up to you to put in the extra effort the next day to work it off, and the chances are it will give you the buzz of a real achievement.

Exercise is the ultimate, flexible option. What you need to do is get your body going so it starts to turn your fat into energy which you then burn up. There are certain *do*'s and *don't*s that will help you keep it up.

- Find a form – or forms – of exercise you can stay with. Fitness needn't involve hours in the gym but it does require consistency, so it's vital to find a pattern that suits you. I know people who have got fit – and lost pounds – from just walking to work. Forty minutes at a good pace is all it takes to feel the benefits. Of course, if your walk to work is boring or depressing, find something else. It may be a gym, a pool, or a cycle ride after work. The important thing is to sustain it.

- After consistency, the second most important thing to remember is to set yourself realistic targets. Don't listen to anyone else: decide what you want to achieve and then go for it. If your goal is weight loss or a general tone-up, make a picture record. Photograph yourself in the same pose and against the same background every week and in a couple of months you'll be amazed at the change in your appearance.

- Make sure you're comfortable. Splash out on a pair of top-flight trainers and kit yourself out with decent clothes such as Gore-Tex or something similar for wet weather, and Lycra to stop chafing. Discomfort mustn't become an excuse.

- Persevere through focusing on your targets and the long term. Getting fit will be hard at first but after a while you'll enjoy the natural high of pushing yourself and if you stop, you'll miss it. Whoever said that about dieting?

- Don't pretend that you can't spare forty five minutes to an hour for your regime. With the good effects of exercise kicking in, you'll be that much more alert and that much quicker. You'll find your day magically expands.

- Do involve other people. A partner will get you going on those mornings when you feel you can't be bothered. Alternatively, think about involving your whole family. Going out together for a bike ride is a great experience. Better still, have everyone set individual targets and then work out a reward scheme for hitting them.

- Don't put it off by saying *I'll join the gym on Monday*. Go for a forty-minute walk. Now.

Fitness has been a big part of my adult life and almost certainly saved it when I was soldiering. But that's not the reason I keep it up. It's not even for the health benefits, although being fit helps all of us live healthier and happier lives.  I do it because I enjoy it and I hope this book can help you enjoy it too.

Good luck!

Chris Ryan
2004

# Introduction

*Chris Ryan talks about physical training and what you will get from his fitness programme*

When I think of fitness I think of something that I can call upon to get me out of a tight spot. I've always needed to use my fitness, as much as I have my soldiering skills and equipment, to keep me out of harm's way. For example, my escape from Iraq in which I covered over 200 miles, walking on my own without any food and with very little water over very harsh terrain. This story was documented in my book, *The One That Got Away*. OK, so your job probably doesn't involve much time spent behind enemy lines but that doesn't mean that you can neglect staying in shape. My maxim applies just as much to you: once you've achieved a good standard of fitness you'll be prepared for anything that's thrown at you.

Of course, I realise that long, boring training programmes are the last thing you want to be saddled with, and that there's nothing more soul-destroying than seeing months and months of graft stretching out in front of you. This is why my programme will see you make significant fitness and strength gains in six weeks and will give you the ability and the motivation to continue indefinitely. You'll probably have to make some lifestyle adjustments in order to make room for your training – and I'll also be asking you to take a look at your diet – but this doesn't mean hard rations from here on in. Nights out on the beer and the occasional curry aren't a thing of the past, and you'll still be able to factor in the things you enjoy because you'll be working hard enough to offset any negative effects they have on your training. All you have to do is stick with it and you'll find that you'll start to enjoy the training and the positive effects that it has on your life. Naturally, this includes looking good – which is a guaranteed by-product of the programme – but this shouldn't be your sole motivation. Because it's about more than just having a body you're not ashamed of; it's about that feeling of quiet

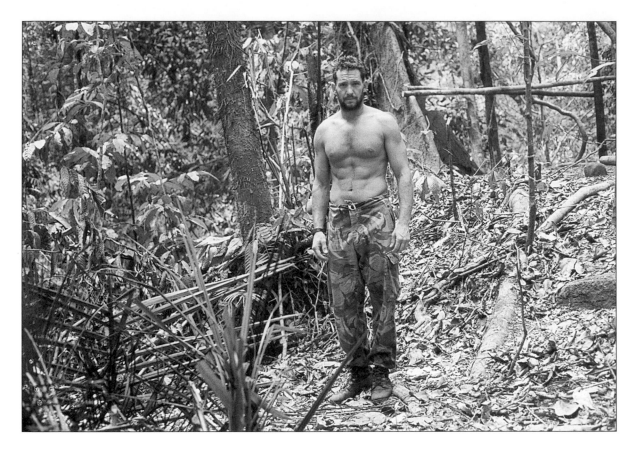

*Even on a 3-month jungle trip, we would make an effort to have an upper-body work out. Note in the top right-hand corner, the horizontal poles on which we would do dips and pull-ups.*

confidence you get when you know you've got what it takes to avoid trouble whenever it tries to pin you down. As well as the aerobic drills and strength circuits you'll find sections on diet, personal kit, dangers and setbacks, warm-ups, cool-downs and stretching. I'll show you how to train safely and effectively ensuring that you do everything you can to avoid injury and get the maximum out of the effort you put in.

I know from my time as an SAS instructor that, even though I was training the cream of the British Army and all the guys under my command maintained an incredibly high standard of physical fitness, some were still in better shape than others. There were guys of all shapes and sizes. That's why my training target was simple: I aimed to exhaust the natural strength of each individual, be it a soldier from the Paras or a Princess. That may sound tough, but it applies to my programme because the only way to make any progress and see improvement is to keep challenging yourself and your body. So whatever level of fitness you're bringing to this book, you'll find drills and exercises that will cut you into great shape because they're all based on quality fitness.

To show you what I mean, let's use as an example those guys who complain that they spend half their lives training without making any great advances. This may even be you. If it is, I can guarantee that the main reason

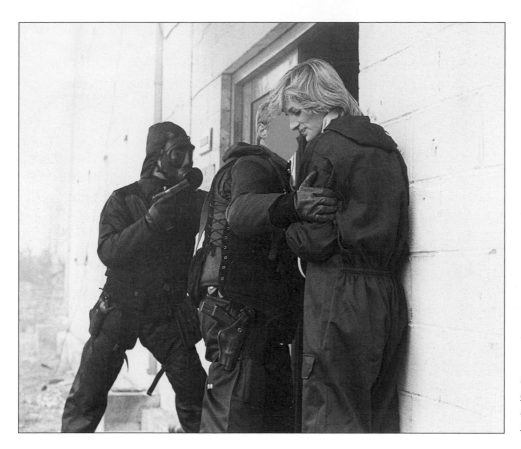

*Princess Diana going into 'the killing house' with SAS members.*

you're not getting anywhere is that you've made time to lift some weights or get out for a run and you're satisfied with that. As long as you put in the hours you're going to get the results. Well, that's rubbish. It's not about how long your workout is, it's about whether you are really pushing yourself during that time. The guys who complain about a lack of results are probably just cruising through their time in the gym. This is a useless attitude, because after a while they give up, pissed off that they aren't feeling any fitness benefits or witnessing any strength gains. But you're never going to get in shape crawling through a workout; you need to push yourself in the aerobic arena and lift progressively heavier weights with good form to see and feel any differences. This is what I mean by quality fitness. If you do this, even the usual excuse – of not having enough time in your day to devote to getting fit – is redundant. If your programme is high in quality you don't have to spend half your life under a bar-bell or in the pool, but can get in and out knowing that you've pushed yourself to the maximum and that your body is already reaping the rewards.

The strength circuits in this book are designed so that you have no choice but to push yourself every week. For the aerobic drills it's a little different, and you're going to rely on a heart-rate monitor (see Personal kit, page 7) to make sure you're exercising at a level where you can guarantee that you're really working the heart and lungs. The heart-rate monitor has completely changed my attitude towards aerobic drills – even though I felt a bit of a fraud at first, because I seemed to be taking it easy compared to what I had been used to in the SAS. Working side by side with the right diet over a period of six to twelve weeks, you can make phenomenal gains without picking up any injuries.

A heart-rate monitor calculates what percentage of its maximum your heart is currently working at. For example, you can get a good aerobic workout by boosting your heart rate to 50 to 60 per cent of its maximum capacity, but you'll need to keep it at that level for well over an hour if you're going to reap any rewards. Better to push yourself harder for a shorter period of time, and boost the intensity of your aerobic drill so that your heart is beating at 70 to 85 per cent of its maximum capacity. Do this, and you can finish your bike ride or run in less time, knowing that you've burned a significant amount of fat and made another step towards peak fitness.

All the aerobic drills in the book have their own training programmes, split into three levels according to your current standard of fitness, and you'll be training between 50 and 85 per cent of your maximum heart-rate for varying amounts of time. You won't be going all out, all the time, particularly if you're new to exercise. What you won't be doing is falling into the trap of exercising at a slow speed over a long period of time. This is so often the recommendation from coaches for weight loss, but exercising like this only slows down the time it takes to see results. This does nothing for the motivation of the individual as they feel that they've have been putting in loads of consistent effort and nothing seems to be happening. And nothing will. After all, if you waltz along at 40 per cent of your maximum effort, you'll burn around two to five calories a minute. Run at the same percentage and you'll burn 7 to 11 calories a minute. Run hard and you'll burn around 20 calories a minute. See the difference.

Ultimately, you've got to assess what your fitness goals are. If it's solely fat reduction then concentrate on the aerobic drills and stick to the level-one strength circuits to keep your muscles toned. If you want to really bulk up and get strong then work though all the levels of the strength circuits, and use any other time you have to do an aerobic drill, so that you can strip away any fat on your body that's hiding those muscles you've worked so hard for.

# 1. Personal kit

## Get your equipment sorted before you go into action

You don't have to spend a fortune on fitness equipment in order to get fit. If you're a member of a gym then all the hardware you need is going to be provided for you; all you've got to worry about are your personal effects. If you're working out at home you can kit yourself out at minimal cost by buying an incline weight bench and a 50kg dumb-bell and bar-bell set.

The bottom line is that if you're not properly prepared for your upcoming fitness campaign, you're just making things more difficult for yourself and that doesn't make sense. You're more likely to be successful if the equipment you're using increases the efficiency of your workout. So take a look at the basic checklist below in which I've detailed the items that can make all the difference.

## Trainers

The toughest part of buying new trainers is looking at the price tag, but if your current pair look like they could degenerate into a pair of flip-flops at any moment, then you really should invest. If your chosen aerobic drill is running, your feet are going to take a pounding. A good pair of trainers can provide you with another important barrier between you and injury. Even if you choose one of the other aerobic drills, the strength circuits require you to have footwear that's going to provide stability and comfort throughout your workout, so you should probably go for a pair of cross trainers. These sit higher up on the foot than running shoes and stabilise your feet throughout a wide range of movement, providing you with good lateral support.

When it comes to running shoes, the most important thing to remember is: if a pair has a three-figure price tag on it, that doesn't mean they're going to protect your feet better than cheaper ones. Forget what the shop assistant is telling you; the person who knows what's best for your feet is you, and as long as you're buying from an informed point of view you can't go wrong.

To do this you first have to know whether your feet are flat, high-arched or normal; so place a piece of cardboard on the bathroom floor and the next time you jump out of the shower or bath, stand on the cardboard then study the imprint left by your feet.

- **HIGH-ARCHED FEET:** If you see narrow bands of flesh connecting the front of your feet with the heels, you have high-arched feet that don't pronate; this means that they don't flex enough and so have trouble absorbing the shock every time they hit the floor. Instead they stay rigid when they hit the ground. You need to go for trainers with a gel-filled chamber under the heel and forefoot, and a polyurethane or spongy EVA mid-sole (between the outer sole and the upper).

- **FLAT FEET:** If the imprint shows all or nearly all of the underside of your foot it means that you're flat-footed. Your feet over-pronate and roll too easily as they hit the floor, which puts a lot of stress on your ankles and arches. You need to look for heavy, rigid trainers with a dual-density mid-sole and stiffer materials in the out-sole.

- **NORMAL FEET:** Anything in between these two means that your feet are normal and they fall on the outside of the heel then roll inward. When you're buying your trainers just make sure that they offer you good support and cushioning.

Whatever kind of feet you have there are some general rules that always apply when you go into the shop to buy your trainers.

First of all, wear the sports socks you would wear during training, and simulate the fact that your feet will swell when you're in the gym by shopping late in the day when your feet swell naturally.

Next, you don't have to cut a trainer open to find out how good its mid-sole is. Instead you can test it by grabbing the heel and toe and flexing it, mimicking the way it will bend when your foot is running in it. If it flexes at the arch then the shoe won't offer you enough rigidity for exercise purposes, so try others until you find one that bends at the ball of the foot.

When you've found a pair that you think is right for you don't be afraid to put them on. But don't just stand in front of a mirror posing, walk or (if possible) run around the shop. Make sure your heel and forefoot fit comfortably without the trainer pinching the skin, and that it's not too tight across the top of your foot. Ensure that there's about a thumbnail's width between your longest toe and the edge of the toe box and that the heel cup doesn't feel too tight, as this can cause problems with your Achilles' tendon. Also, don't forget that you can fine-tune the comfort of your trainer with inserts like heel cups, pads, and full- and half-length insoles.

## Heart-rate monitor

As I've already explained in the introduction, this gadget is absolutely vital for quality fitness, and to ensure that during your aerobic workouts you're always operating as efficiently as possible. No longer the preserve of marathon runners, a heart-rate monitor is finally being recognised as a cheap, digitised personal trainer and an essential piece of kit. It consists of a transmitter and a wrist receiver, and all you have to do is adjust the transmitter so that it fits snugly around your chest, then wet the grooved electrode areas on the back of it to make sure that your heart-rate transmissions are as clear as possible. The wrist receiver will pick up your heart rate and show it on the read-out as a percentage of its maximum. This will allow you to train at a pace that will give you maximum benefit in terms of weight loss and cardiovascular fitness.

There are a lot of models out there and prices vary. Polar is a very popular brand, and top sports labels like Nike are launching their own versions, which is proof of how established they are as a fitness tool. Just make sure that you get one that measures and displays heart rate with ECG precision.

## Waterproof jacket

In our climate it's nearly always pissing down – which is just another excuse to talk yourself out of your aerobic drill. So get a loose-fitting jacket that's made from breathable fabric like Sympatex, which will allow body moisture to evaporate while keeping you dry when it rains.

## Waterproof pants

One disadvantage of wearing long waterproof pants is that you have a tendency to sweat and overheat. A good idea therefore for the bottoms is to wear long Lycra running pants. These will keep your legs warm in harsh conditions because the Lycra draws the sweat away from the skin.

## *Lycra shorts*

If you aren't used to cross-terrain walking, running or cycling, Lycra shorts are essential because they will stop any chafing around your groin area. I know from experience how important they are: on one occasion I went for a run around town with some guys from the regiment after coming back from a long trip abroad during which I hadn't been doing any running at all. I went out without Lycra shorts because they were still thought of as women's sportswear by the other guys, and you were liable to have the mickey taken out of you. I instantly regretted it though – I chafed so badly on a ten-miler that I was actually bleeding by the time I made it back. It was absolute agony. After that I didn't care how much of a ribbing I got.

Thankfully, Lycra is now accepted sportswear, so whether you're going out for a walk or a run put some on. If you don't feel comfortable in them in terms of what they look like, just wear a pair of baggy shorts on top.

# 2. Diet

## *Back up your training with the right kind of fuel*

Behind every layer of fat there are toned muscles trying to get out, and if you're not eating the right kind of food to underpin your fitness programme, then a lot of your effort will go unnoticed – particularly around your belly. You need to realise that training is not restricted to the gym and the bike, but continues when you get home and open your fridge.

The first thing you need to do is look at your fat intake, especially if your local curry house sends you a Christmas card every year. It's recommended that our daily intake of fat should be restricted to 90g. If you're trying to lose weight you should be looking to halve this.

Within the 90g guideline we should have no more than 31g of saturated fats. These are the ones that are solid at room temperature, e.g. butter, or the fat round a pork chop. Saturated fats will not only add to the size of your waistline but will also raise your cholesterol level.

There's fat in just about everything you eat. But you can't live your life without it, so just try to look for daily opportunities to cut it out of your diet and incorporate some of the following strategies when buying, cooking or eating food.

- Whenever you can, grill, bake, poach, boil or steam as an alternative to frying. If you have no choice then make sure you use a non-stick pan to cut down on the added fat. If you're frying an egg, for example, you only have to add a drop of oil to a heated non-stick pan, and then roll it around. Even better to ditch your bottle of cooking oil and buy a low-fat spray. The most careful pouring of oil will add around 15g of fat to the meal, a spray will add only 1g per shot.
- Go easy when you're applying butter or margarine to toast. You can either spread it thinly or use none at all under beans or jam; you'll hardly notice the difference.

- Always look for the leanest cuts of meat, but be aware that even lean cuts will require some trimming to get rid of all the fat. The best way to do this is to place the cut in the freezer for half an hour first. You'll find that all the fat will turn white, making it easier for you to identify and cut off.
- Use low-fat mayonnaise wherever possible.
- Use skimmed milk for cooking, especially sauces that call for large amounts of milk, cream and butter. Dishes made from skimmed or semi-skimmed milk aren't that much different from those made from whole milk. Substitute a cup of skimmed milk for a cup of cream and you're cutting 60 calories out of the recipe straight away. Alternatively, you can use low-fat yogurt or fromage frais.
- Make salad dressings from natural yogurt, herbs, spices, tomato juice, vinegar or lemon juice.
- Buy skinless chicken or turkey. About half the fat you'll find in poultry is either in or directly under the skin.
- Dry fry mincemeat, and pour off the fat as it melts.
- Use half-fat hard cheese, cottage cheese or, if you have to, very small portions of stronger flavoured full-fat cheese.
- Eat more beans and less meat and you'll get all the protein you need and a lot less fat.
- When you buy canned tuna buy it packed in brine or water instead of oil, which adds a significant amount of fat to the meat.
- Substitute those mid-afternoon high-fat snacks like crisps or chocolates for a carbohydrate rich, low-fat fruit bun or scone.
- Turn yourself into a compulsive label reader when you're in the supermarket; it's the only way to be completely sure that you're cutting back on fat. To qualify as low-fat the meal must contain less than 5g of fat per 100g, so if you see something marked 'light', 'lite', 'reduced fat', or 'lower-fat' don't sling it in your basket automatically. Products labelled like this only have to have 25 per cent less fat than normal.
- Get into the habit of placing a couple of dishes of vegetables on the table for every meal and always be within reach of a bowl of fruit. This gives you even less of an excuse to fill up on fatty foods – and for every bite of vegetable or fresh fruit there's less room for steak-and-kidney pie or cheesecake.

Of course you're not always going to be in a position to dictate what you eat and how it's cooked, but I still have a few tricks that mean I can have a night out without piling on loads of weight.

**At the cinema:** Don't have salted popcorn, there's about 45g of fat in a 100g serving. Sweet popcorn isn't much better with 20g of fat per 100g. Have wine gums or fruit pastilles instead, which contain only a trace of fat.

**At the restaurant:** Have your vegetables without butter, and coffee with milk and not cream. These two insignificant changes will knock 20g of fat off your meal's total.

**At the curry house:** Swap your beef kheema and naan for chicken tikka and rice. You'll save at least 70g of fat.

**At the pizza place:** Skip the garlic bread and save yourself the equivalent of at least a tablespoon of butter, then blot the top of your pizza with a paper serviette before you eat it to save around 4.5g of fat per slice.

**At the Chinese take-away:** Leave the last half-inch of your meal in the container. By eating only the top of the food you get all the meat and vegetables but leave the fat in the foil.

**At the kebab shop:** Go for a chicken shish kebab which is basically grilled, skewered chicken in a plain pitta filled with salad and contains, on average, only 10g of fat. This really is the healthy option compared to the traditional doner kebab which packs at least 50g of fat.

**At the burger bar:** Go for a flame-grilled burger and ask them to hold the mayonnaise and you're looking at only around 12g of fat.

If you're trying to bulk up, the key is to base your meals around good quality protein – egg white, chicken, meat, fish – to maintain and repair the muscles after every workout, and include fruit and vegetables at every opportunity to supply the essential micro nutrients. All you need to do then is add some carbohydrates, like bread, rice, pasta and potatoes, which fuel the muscles.

The only problem can be that your diet can degenerate into a series of bland meals if you don't know how to spice things up a little, and it's vital that things still taste good if you're going to stick to a diet throughout your programme. For most guys there are just three seasonings: butter, salt and pepper, but you'll be amazed at what you can do if you spend some time at the spice rack. Go for spice blends and keep things simple by having one for red meat, one for chicken, one for fish and one for vegetables.

There's also a lot of help around for the low-fat cook these days in terms of recipe books and magazines which will provide you with hundreds of tasty meals that are low in fat and geared to specific goals. Alternatively, supermarkets have their own low-fat range of produce and ready-to-eat meals – although don't take it for granted that it's low in fat until you've read the label.

I take advantage of both – and like baking a skinless chicken breast in foil with grated pepper and some lemon, eating it with wholemeal pasta or rice (because that kind of carbohydrate burns more slowly inside you). I also use fresh tuna or even mince up a turkey breast, then add some chopped chillies, onion, an egg white, breadcrumbs and pepper, and shape it into a couple of burgers that you can put on a tray and bake. These are great with wholemeal pitta bread and salad.

★　　★　　★

When it comes to alcohol I'm no saint, but you need to try and steer clear as much as you can. Drinking three ounces of alcohol reduces the body's ability to burn fat one-third. And if you've been out on the beer all night you're not going to be able to train effectively; you're leaving yourself more prone to dehydration too. And of course alcohol is extremely high in calories, which get converted into simple sugars – and that means fat. A pint of beer contains 200 calories, and that's nearly as much as a Snickers bar.

So you need to count beer as part of your calorie intake, but don't cheat on food so that you can drink more beer. Alcohol has few, if any, nutrients and inhibits the absorption of nutrients from the food you do eat, so drinking on an empty stomach will just bring on your cravings and you'll end up snacking on crisps, nuts and kebabs.

If you've got a particular weight-loss goal then you should try and give up for a while – drive to the dinner party and you won't have any choice but to stay off the booze. But if you're using my programme to stay fit for life, then just try to drink in moderation.

# 3. Dangers and setbacks

## *Your training can be ambushed at any time, so know your enemies*

No training plan is going to go completely without a hitch so you need to know how to cope with the things that can derail your programme. When a regiment guy wasn't training it was because he had broken his arm or his leg, and even then you'd still see him in the gym with his plaster pushing weight on the part of his body that wasn't broken. I wouldn't recommend this, however, you do need to know how to keep certain dangers at bay or how to deal with them when they hit.

## *Dehydration*

I've seen the effects of extreme dehydration at close quarters, and it's not pretty. During the first contact we had in the Gulf one of the lads had his thermals on because he hadn't had a chance to change out of them when we were compromised by the enemy. During the hectic, 45-minute fire-fight that ensued, the amount of body fluid he lost as sweat put him down as soon as the adrenalin had stopped flowing. That man was a rower and one of the strongest guys in the regiment, but dehydration had taken him out of the game completely. You've got to make sure that the same thing doesn't happen to you. The longer and harder you push your body the more you're going to need to drink. That's fact, and if you think it doesn't apply to you then it won't be long before we're going to have to casevac (casualty evacuation) you from the treadmill.

When you work hard during your aerobic drills or strength training circuits your muscles generate heat, and it's this heat that burns your calories and fries your fat. Around 70 per cent of this heat needs to escape from the body – to avoid cooking you alive from the inside out. It does this in the form of sweat, which evaporates from your skin and takes the unwanted heat with it. However, if you don't replace this fluid loss your blood thickens and your heart has to work harder to move it through the bloodstream, thus slowing the delivery of oxygen and nutrients to your muscles. This results in a loss of work-rate, fatigue and, if you let it go too far, more serious repercussions. Just look at the following table, which shows the physical effects of dehydration expressed as a percentage.

- **1 per cent dehydration** You'll feel thirsty.
- **2 per cent dehydration** You'll feel parched and will experience a loss of appetite and, unknown to you, a 20 per cent reduction in your capacity for exercise.
- **4 per cent dehydration** Tiredness, nausea and emotional instability will kick in.
- **6 per cent dehydration** You'll start to lose colour and will probably experience waves of acute nausea, aggressiveness and irritability.
- **10 per cent dehydration** Very severe symptoms present themselves and your thermoregulation systems start breaking down, leaving you unable to regulate body temperature.
- **11 per cent dehydration** Sometime soon you're going to need urgent medical assistance to restore the chemical imbalances that are going on in your body. Someone needs to rehydrate you very quickly.
- **20 per cent dehydration** You've reached the limits of what the body can take.
- **21 per cent dehydration** You're off to that big drinking fountain in the sky.

The best way to make sure none of this happens to you is to know how to prehydrate and rehydrate efficiently, no matter what exercise you're doing.

A good way to work out your state of hydration is to start weighing yourself before and after exercise. Any weight loss experienced straight after your workout probably won't be lost from your fat reserves; it's more likely to be due to water loss, and you should replenish every pound you've lost by drinking 750ml of water. Of course, you can pre-empt the water loss that you will experience by prehydrating a few hours before your workout in anticipation of the fluid loss. Do this by drinking half a litre of water, then follow the guidelines set out in the table below showing how much fluid you should be drinking during each of the performance exercises in this book.

- **Cross-terrain walking (1 day with Bergen*)**  Drink 4 litres
- **Running (10 km)**  Drink 500ml to 700ml
- **Cycling (1 hour)**  Drink 700ml to 750ml
- **Swimming (45 minutes)**  Drink 300ml

- Rowing (45 minutes)                    Drink 300ml to 400ml
- Strength training circuit (1 hour)     Drink 250ml

(* an army-issue haversack)

Obviously, it's difficult to keep hydrated during drills like swimming and rowing, so you should ensure that when you finish you drink at least 250ml to 500ml of water. Remember to drink past the feeling of thirst, since this is just a sensation that shuts down once you've taken a few mouthfuls. Psychologically your thirst has been quenched, but physically your body is crying out for more water and is still dehydrated. If you're not drinking from a bottle and are dependent on a water fountain in a gym, you can still judge how much water you're taking on by counting your swallows. The average, full-mouth swallow contains about 15ml of liquid, although when you're bent over drinking from a water fountain it's a little less at around 10ml per gulp.

You're not limited to water to keep you hydrated; there are a number of sports drinks on the market that claim to do the job much more effectively. In reality, you'll need to be really going some in order to make use of the beneficial effects of a sports drink: if you've been training really hard for 90 minutes or more, sports drinks can supply you with the kind of quick calories required for consistent performance (around 60 to 100 calories per 150ml); if you're working out at the levels in this book, even though they are by no means easy, it's not really necessary to replace the loss in sodium, potassium and other electrolytes. You won't deplete your body's natural reserves to anything like a dangerous level. Only if you progress from this programme to something like an Ironman competition should you start thinking about sports drinks.

## Plateauing

The reason that all the aerobic drills and weight circuits in this book have motivation sections is to break you loose from that non-productive phase that everyone who sticks with a fitness programme experiences. Your muscles and fitness level should continually be in a state of progression, and in order to do this you have to keep them constantly challenged.

It's all too easy to fall into the trap of doing the same workout every week, for months on end. Instead, you should look to shake up your workout, on average, every three to six weeks. Because even though you will experience plenty of benefits to begin with, after a while the rewards will become less noticeable as your body is stressed in the same way again and again and your muscle fibres adapt. You will either stop noticing any differences in your body shape, or will get through your chosen aerobic exercise without breaking sweat. This is called a plateau, and you will experience them at every level – so the quicker you learn how to kick-start your programme the better.

The important thing here is constantly to adjust your aerobic drills or weight circuits when you find that you're not getting any increased benefits. The first line of attack against an aerobic plateau is to increase the amount of time you spend in your target heart-rate zone, perhaps by two minutes per week.

You can do this by occasionally going faster with interval training or 'pyramids' (examples of which I've included in all the aerobic sections). To give you an idea, interval training involves increasing your effort from the pace you would normally walk, run, cycle, swim or row for a short period of time, then dropping back to the normal pace, repeating this speed/recovery cycle a number of times. Pyramids are similar, in that you build up your pace incrementally, for a particular period of time, until you reach a target, when you bring the pace back down until you're back where you started. If you're on an aerobic drill that involves terrain (walking, running, cycling), then you can do hill work to shake up your programme. For example, if you're running near a slope but not actually utilising it, do so, running up the hill two to five times depending on what level of fitness you're at.

When it comes to the strength training circuits, the only way you're going to develop body strength is to rely on the intensity of your workout. To do this you have to overload it with increasingly heavier resistance. If you can't lift the last one or two repetitions of a set with good form it's not a bad thing, it's an indication that your circuit set is exactly right. You've got to be constantly thinking about lifting more weight and never be satisfied to cruise through your repetitions without feeling a twinge in your muscles.

However, to go forward you sometimes have to go backwards first – and this couldn't be truer than with the plateau you will experience with strength training. To get your muscles to lift more weight you often have to trick them by tinkering with the way you lift weight. Here are some tried and tested examples:

● **Active rest:** Try mixing exhaustive stretches of training with planned periods of active rest. For example, if you can't seem to get past a certain weight on the bench press, drop the number of sets you're doing by one and cut the weight by about 70 per cent for your first workout. For the remaining workouts in the week gradually build the weight back to your starting point, adding more on each set until you're back where you started. These active rest periods allow full recovery of the muscles while keeping them used to the process of lifting weight, and should mean that your last workout of the week should see you breaking your weight barrier.

- **Slow it down:** Taking longer over the lift itself can result in an improvement, because the targeted muscles are being stressed for longer. In one study two groups of weightlifters were compared. One group trained by taking seven seconds over a repetition (two seconds up, one second hold, four seconds down), while the other group took 14 seconds (ten seconds up and four seconds down). The slow-lifting group was found to be stronger after two months.
- **Cut the repetitions:** For example, from ten to eight – but lifting more weight.
- **Use a spotter:** Get someone to spot for you and either do negative or forced repetitions. The first means that your spotter helps you lift a weight that's heavier than you could ordinarily handle, while you control the weight on your own as you lower it. Forced repetitions come at the end of a set, when you've reached failure – this is when your spotter helps you to do two or three more repetitions. If you do use a spotter make sure that you tell them exactly what you want so that, when you get to the sticking point (that crucial moment on the last few repetitions where you're struggling to lift the weight), they don't just grab the bar and start working it for you. Brief them that you still want to do the work, they're just there to help you if you get into trouble with the weight after failure.
- **Pyramids:** Do a pyramid by lifting progressively heavier weights with each set. By adding a little more weight to each set you can trick your muscles into going beyond the point where they would normally be fatigued. For example, if you're doing some dumb-bell curls, start with a slightly lighter weight than you would normally lift on your first set. Curl them five times, take a short rest, then add more weight, but still not your maximum, and do five more repetitions. Continue in this way until you reach a weight that you fail to curl five times and you'll probably find that you've lifted a heavier weight than you would usually. Now work your way back down the weights. Do this for a few workouts and you'll find that you will, most likely, have left your plateau behind.
- **Cut the weight:** Occasionally switch to lighter weights and increase the repetitions.
- **Reverse pyramids:** Go heavy-to-light with a reverse pyramid that starts with your heaviest weight for a few repetitions, then a lighter weight for a few more repetitions, and so on, until you finish with approximately 12 repetitions using a light weight. In doing this your muscles lift the heaviest weight when they're freshest, so you can often do more repetitions with the heavy weight than you would have done had you had lifted it when your muscles were exhausted.

- **Switch it:** If you normally do your aerobic drill before your weight circuits, do it afterwards instead. This way your body learns to work through different levels of fatigue.
- **Substitution:** Swap one exercise for another – substitute dumb-bells for bar-bells, or an incline bench press for a flat one. Return to the original exercise after about three weeks.
- **Change your grips:** For example, underhand for overhand, or close for wide. Just make sure you're not working the same muscle from the same angle for two exercises in a row.

## Overtraining

This has affected me twice in my life, at both ends of my time with the SAS. Overtraining (or burnout) is like a disease, and the first time I experienced it I was training for selection. I used to run 10 miles to the swimming baths, do a mile in the pool, run home, and then do 16 miles on my bike – every night for three months. I started to get sleepless nights, became irritable and lacked concentration. I found that I was picking up loads of injuries which I was just training through and compounding, making them worse, until one day my body just couldn't take it any more and I found myself in all sorts of trouble. In effect, I had to go cold turkey from training until I got back to normal and had given my body a chance to recover.

The second example came when I had been with the regiment for eight years. I was put on training wing as one of the instructors who handles selection. I knew I had to get myself fitter than I had been eight years earlier (when I had gone for it myself) because I was going to be up against young guys determined to get in. I was looking forward to it, however, because I now knew the dangers of overtraining. I started the process of walking, running and getting my Bergen on my back and going up and down Pen-y-Fan, so that when selection started I was really able to beast all the young lads and get the best out of them.

We went to the jungle and I did the same: leading from the front with my Bergen, doing advance-to-contact training and combat survival. But by the time I'd finished with this first wave of selection the next lot was just about to start – so I had to go through the whole process again. I found that my body had been breaking down through the intensity of the first selection and I hadn't had enough time to recover, repair and build it back up.

By the time I came on to the third selection I was under immense pressure to perform and my body was beginning to really suffer. I could see that my plan to come back super-fit wasn't going to work out – and the rumour that you always came back from training wing absolutely wasted was true. During the fourth selection wave I broke my ankle free-falling, which gave my body a chance to rest.

What these examples demonstrate is that overtraining can affect you whether you know about it or not, so set yourself realistic goals and work to each goal with the required amount of rest and recovery. When you start really getting into your programme, particularly at level three, and you see the positive effects that it's having on your body, it's natural to think that more is better and to neglect your rest days and recovery periods. Take it from me, your body needs to rest, and if you continually beast it without remorse you will burnout after about two weeks and you'll fall flat on your face because your body won't have anything left to give.

## Schedule

One of the biggest obstacles to sticking with an exercise programme is finding the time to fit it in around your life. Very few of us can afford the luxury of spending the amount of time we would like on our programmes, and there are always going to be times when we don't think we've got time to train. But, as I suggested in the introduction, as long as you keep the emphasis on quality fitness and employ the following techniques when you're pushed for time, it shouldn't be a major problem.

- **Split circuits:** These make up the bulk of the strength circuits which means that when you step up to level two and you're working out around four times a week, the workouts don't take for ever so you can hit your muscles hard and fast and still be able to get on with your life. If you can fit in your aerobic exercise without disrupting your spare time, i.e. by running in the park at lunchtime or cycling to work, then you've got one less excuse for giving up on your programme.
- **Compound exercises:** A lot of the exercises in the weight circuits are compound exercises, which hit several large muscle groups in one shot. Compound exercises are great because they're like doing three or four exercises at once. Examples are the simple dumb-bell row which works most of the muscles in the back and shoulders and the biceps; or the leg press which works the quadriceps, calves, hamstrings and rear.
- **Rest periods:** If you're doing an upper-body circuit one day and a lower-body circuit the next, you'll need to rest between exercises to give your muscles a chance to recover. However, if you alternate upper-body exercises with lower-body exercises within a circuit, then you can cut out recovery time completely and drastically reduce the length of time your workout takes. This is called circuit training, and by switching between

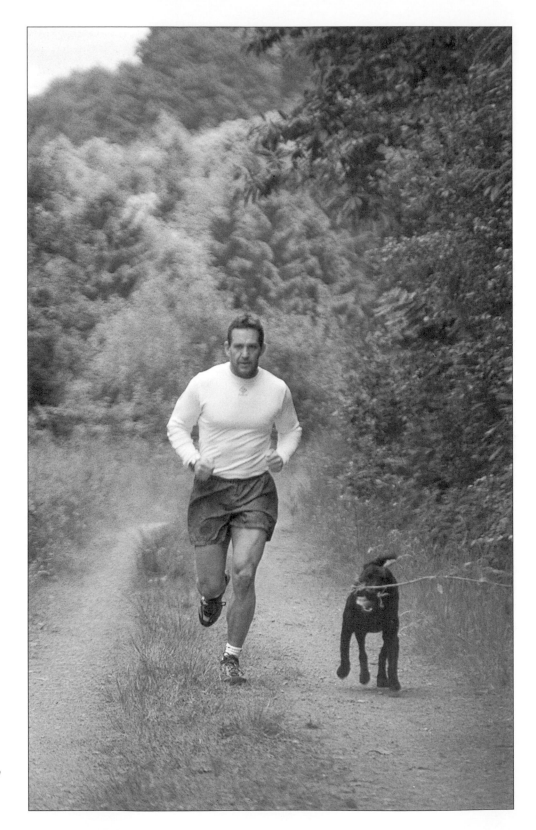

*Out running with my training partner.*

upper-body and lower-body exercises it allows you to rest one set of muscles as you work on a completely different set. All you have to do is take half an upper-body workout and splice it together with half a lower-body workout, then do the other halves the next time you work out. Not only does this kind of training allow you to squeeze a maximum amount of exercise into the minimum amount of time but it also means that you will keep your heart rate elevated at a respectable level throughout, and so improve your cardiovascular abilities as well.

## Boredom

I know what a powerful enemy boredom can be. On the third day of my escape from Iraq I had to lay up in a hollow among some loose rocks in a wadi. If I moved I knew that the risk of capture increased dramatically. But there was nothing alive in the desert to keep me interested, no birds or animals. It took all my will power to resist the urge to move on, or even to just have a look round.

Boredom is a significant reason why most people give up on their exercise programmes. Long, hard workouts take their toll on you psychologically as well as physically, and you have to be really tough to keep up the intensity of your workout, even for a month. The advantage of my higher intensity, quality-fitness workout is that your workout is never the same. You are constantly pushing it to different levels and mixing it up, and as a result you see and feel the effects much more quickly. There's no greater motivational tool than seeing the results of your workout as your body gets cut down to shape and you feel fitter and healthier.

Another way to beat boredom is to get yourself a training partner, someone who has similar goals to yourself who is going to keep you motivated when you feel like skipping training. They don't even have to be human. My training partner is my dog, and I know I've got to walk him every day. He's always happy, he'll walk or run, and he's always on call.

# 4. The warm-up and cool-down

## Don't think you're the one guy who can get away without them – you can't

Going into action 'cold' is something that I had to get used to in the regiment. I usually didn't have the luxury of making sure my body was prepared for the stresses and rigours that I was about to put it through, I just had to get on and do a job. You couldn't complain that you had a twinge or a strain just before you were about to jump through a window. I've seen guys run up hills, jump over a wall into a building, shoot at a couple of people and climb down a rope, and only complain afterwards that they've been carrying pulled muscles, strains, knocks and sometimes even gunshot wounds. For us there was little you could do but absorb the pain and stick it out. But given the luxury of some time and an absence of gunfire (I'll presume you have both) I'll always warm up before running, swimming, jumping on a bike or hitting the weight bench.

However, I do realise that time is one of the greatest obstacles on the route to total fitness. Like me, most of you can't afford to spend half your lives warming up before getting on with your aerobic training, so do what I do and incorporate your warm-up into whatever aerobic drill you've chosen to do. For example, if I'm in the pool I'll tag a warm-up on to the start – before I begin really going for it, I'll do 100 metres of breaststroke, 400 metres of crawl and 100 metres of backstroke, to make sure all the different muscle groups I'm about to put under stress have been warmed up. And this works for whatever discipline you've chosen. Whether you're walking, running, cycling, swimming or rowing, just go at a comfortable pace for ten minutes before you kick into a higher gear. When it comes to weight training, you should warm up on a bike or a rower before you begin lifting. The fact remains that if you're serious about getting fit, then you need to get serious about your warm-up as well, or else you're going to shock your body into action when it's not ready.

If you're still not convinced about a warm-up's legitimacy in your fitness programme, here's what current intelligence tells us about its benefits:

- By increasing your body temperature, a warm-up softens your body and prepares your skeletal muscle for the stress it's about to be put under during exercise.
- It sends a warning to your heart that it'll need to start stepping up a gear. A warm-up ensures that the heart and blood vessels are given time to adjust to the increased demand for oxygen that comes through intensive exercise. This increase in blood to the heart reduces the risk of cardiac abnormalities.
- The increased level of blood reaching your muscles helps deliver fuels, such as glucose, which are vital for energy production. Increased blood saturation of your muscles, tendons and ligaments increases their elasticity, so any movement during exercise can be performed more safely and effectively. This decrease in muscle viscosity means that they perform with more efficiency and power during your workout.
- It wakes up nerve impulses, so co-ordination improves, resulting in a better performance of motor tasks during weight training.
- A warm-up simply prepares the muscles and acts as a transition period from a state of rest to a state of heavy exercise, so there is less chance of muscle soreness afterwards.

You should always end an aerobic drill by cooling down, which doesn't have to be any more hassle than your warm-up. It simply entails an easing-off period during which your heart rate remains consistently below the level of exertion that it was under during the main part of the training section. This is the period when you have to begin refilling the physical reserves of energy that you've used up during exercise, achieving something called super-compensation.

It's during a cool-down that we can actually increase our body's storage capacity for energy, so that the next time we train aerobically there is potentially more energy available to us, i.e. we are fitter.

At the end of a really hard workout the chemical processes responsible for preparing more energy in the muscle cells cease to operate, which is the reason we get knackered and feel we can't carry on. This is when lactic acid floods the muscles because the body can no longer meet its demand for oxygen. The reason that a cool-down is so essential at this point, rather than just collapsing in a heap on the floor for half an hour, is that it encourages increased circulation in the muscles you've been working, which delivers more oxygen via the bloodstream which continues to process the lactic acid. With a comprehensive cool-down, enough oxygen will be made available to extract all the energy from the lactic acid, and we increase our ability to build up greater energy reserves. The lactic acid then ends up as water and carbon dioxide, which are filtered and expelled via the lungs and urine rather than causing you discomfort and muscle soreness.

Finish your cool down with a few stretches, which will take only a few minutes. These are ideal after a workout because they will reduce the tension your muscles have been under, and you'll be stretching them when they are warm and at their most pliable. Stretching also aids circulation and helps to break down the by-products of aerobic exercise; helping you to feel more relaxed, which encourages a swifter and more efficient recovery process.

# 5. Cross-terrain walking

## It's time to get serious about your strolls

When I was back in Hereford after the Gulf, I worked out the exact distances I had walked to avoid detection during my time in the Iraqi desert. The furthest I'd walked in one march before then was the 65 kilometres that made up the final march on selection. But after just the first night, before and after the patrol split, I'd already covered 70 kilometres. By the end of my walk I'd covered a total of 290 kilometres, or just under 200 miles.

My ability to keep moving under the cover of night, even when all my muscles were screaming out for rest, meant the difference between freedom and capture. But if I'd attempted my break for the Syrian border at anything other than a fast march I doubt I would have made it because my body wouldn't have held together over that distance. Of course, I wouldn't recommend anything as extreme as 290 kilometres in a week for aerobic exercise but, as my experience showed, walking is an aerobic drill that places the minimal amount of strain on the body during movement.

For example, when you run, you put pressure on your joints equal to three to five times your own body weight, but when you walk this strain is reduced to only one and a half times your body weight. Therefore, if you're not used to pounding away on a treadmill or you've got back problems or trouble with your hip, knee or ankle joints, it's best to choose walking as a starting point for your aerobic drills.

Walking is the best way to ease yourself into an eventual running programme, which is the natural progression for the exercise. For example, starting with 45 minutes of walking three to four times a week will soon lead to an increase in the pace you walk for those 45 minutes, and eventually you'll feel that you are ready and willing to break into a light jog for the same amount of time. The other great advantage is that it really is whole-body training, incorporating a huge number of muscle groups in the reach and impact phases. In fact, a study on walking, published in the journal *Sports*

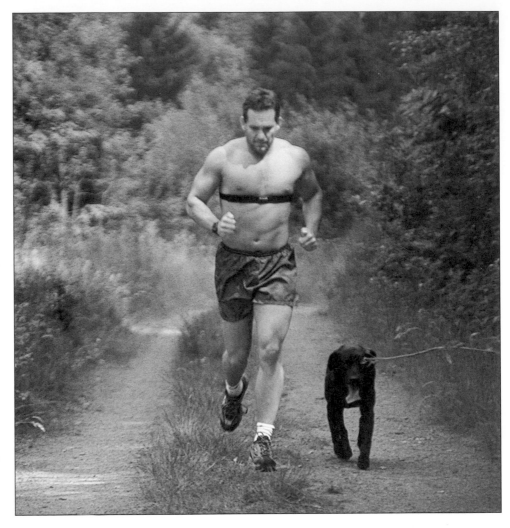

*Using the heart-rate monitor is the best way to train at your selected heart-rate intensity.*

*Medicine*, concluded that 'walking is the activity which comes the closest to being the perfect exercise'. Every day I try to do a walk on my heart-rate monitor, for a minimum of an hour; even when I'm working on my level-three strength circuits I will go for a walk on my rest day. But before you set off anywhere, let me give you a few marching orders.

## Technique

Of course, you've been walking for most of your life so it's a little redundant for me to go into pages of explanation here. However, that doesn't mean your technique and posture is perfect while you're walking; it's probably quite the opposite in fact, because in your lifetime's worth of walking you've probably picked up a lifetime's worth of bad habits without even realising it. And these are bad habits that need straightening out before you start, so troubleshoot your technique by looking at the following table before you begin.

- **UPPER BODY:** Straighten your torso out and tighten your stomach. The number of guys who walk like someone twice their age amazes me, so relax your shoulders and push out your chest. This means that your shoulder blades will automatically slot into the best position. Imagine that you're carrying two moderately heavy bags of shopping in either hand as a rough guide. Your head should form the natural extension of your spine and you should always look on ahead of you, at a distance of around 10 metres.

- **ARMS:** Keep your arms close to your body, with your upper and lower arms forming a fairly sharp angle with one another (the faster you walk the sharper the angle will be). Swing them in a natural rhythm at the sides of your body, but don't swing them too erratically; they should never go above chest height on the upswing or behind your hip bone on the back-swing. Hold your hands in a loose fist.

- **LEGS:** First off, don't think about taking huge steps all the time, walk naturally. Your heel should strike the ground first then the rest of the whole foot to the toes. Make a conscious effort to push off from the ground as you go from one stride into the next and ensure your knees are slightly flexed as you go from one stride into the next.

- **BREATHING:** As long as you're walking as instructed breathing won't be a problem as it will be unrestricted and natural. If you do find that you're short of breath (and you haven't really been pushing yourself hard) check your body position remembering, most importantly, to open up your chest. Correct breathing should have you breathing in deeply, but not like you're actively trying to fill your lungs. If you find that you're taking shallow breaths then think about inhaling over the first three to four steps and exhaling over the next three or four.

## Fat-burning

Walking has never been thought of as an efficient fat-burning activity, but performed at the right intensity for the right length of time it can shift excess weight as effectively as running. You'll be able to boost your heart rate to 50 to 60 per cent of its maximum capacity while walking, but because this isn't particularly high you'll need to keep it at that level for 45 minutes to an hour to get any real fitness and fat-burning benefits; but you should be able to do this pretty easily because of the low-impact nature of the exercise. For this reason you'll find that beginner walkers lose even more fat than beginner joggers, who'll probably be knackered after 10 minutes and stop before they've been able to get into their target zone for fat-burning. This is why walking can be a really effective exercise. In fact, 'power walking' at a moderate pace can burn 600 calories an hour, more than jogging at a moderate pace. This is because, unlike running, you're utilising most of your upper body as well. Here are a few tips on 'power walking' technique.

- Swing your arms back behind your body but keep them relaxed at all times. Tensing your arms just wastes energy.
- Keep your back straight because if you power walk with a bent back the stress of the walk will be absorbed by improperly aligned body parts and this will take its toll on your back and knees.
- Make sure your hips move forward and back, not side to side, because you want all your body to be moving forward so that you don't waste any momentum and reduce the efficiency of the power walk.

Even if power walking isn't hardcore enough for you and you'd rather be running, don't completely dismiss a walk because it can help you make those high-intensity runs all the more productive (see Running, page 31).

To turn your walk into an even more effective calorie-burner you can load up a Bergen or rucksack and take that out with you. We were often saddled with huge individual loads during operations; the average weight of our Bergens was around 60 kilos, and that's not including a belt-kit of pouches weighing around 20 kilos. With that lot on you had to walk with your head down like a donkey most of the time, and if you fell on your back you'd have a hard job getting up. The loads were so heavy that they pulled out any stitches you had in, and someone else had to help you on with them. I'm not suggesting that you damage yourself by packing a rucksack full of breeze-blocks (especially if you have a weak back), so don't go out with a rucksack of more than 50lbs. Although it may have felt fine in your living room, by the time you've climbed that first hill you'll realise how much weight it is. Just be aware that the heavier your rucksack is, the heavier you will be, and the more calories your body will burn at every step.

The surface you're walking on will also dictate how much fat you're burning. For example, walking on sand burns up twice the calories of a road. Don't wimp out of taking on a hill as this obviously requires more effort than walking on a flat surface. Walking slowly up a steep hill will burn as many calories as running on flat ground, and if you're going at around 5mph then walking up a moderate incline can burn anywhere from 10 to 15 calories a minute. Walk into the wind when you can as well, because air resistance is an excellent fat burner. Ultimately, you need to remember to keep the pace up. I'm used to going very, very fast – tabbing or speed marching without running, probably at a speed of nine kilometres an hour. So always push yourself to walk faster, because the faster your walking speed the less efficient you get at it, ensuring that the energy you burn is much greater.

## Motivation

The more you can vary the difficulty of your walk the better, because it can get very monotonous very quickly if the scenery isn't up to much. There are quite a few tricks you can employ to stay on track, and a good place to start is by altering the speed of your walk. Try walking pyramids, for example; go hard for a minute, then slow it down for a minute, go hard for two minutes, slower for two minutes, hard for three minutes, easy for three minutes, then after a while work back down again so that you finish your workout with the above intervals in reverse order. If you're not sure how fast you're going, here's a well-known guide to determine at what speed you're walking, devised by the US cardiologist Dr James Rippe who first coined the term 'fitness walking'.

- **20 minutes a mile (3 mph):** The speed you would walk around at work.
- **15 minutes a mile (4 mph):** Brisk walking, when you're late for an appointment.
- **12 minutes a mile (5 mph):** A determined, brisk pace.

Another thing you can do to break up the monotony and maintain quality fitness throughout your walking session is to go off-road. Always try to walk cross-terrain where possible, because the more uneven the ground, the harder it is to push off from it and the more energy is needed to travel across it. Another great motivational tool that I used to employ was reducing a huge walk into manageable stages. So if I was on the hills with my Bergen I would look ahead and find a target to walk to, e.g. a small clump of bushes, then when I got there I'd take a few breaths and say to myself, right, I'm going to walk to the ridge line. In this way you split up a hard, taxing walk into stages that are easier to handle.

## Training

- **LEVEL ONE:** If you start at this level then you should be training two to three times a week. Start with a 10- to 15-minute walk, then build up to 45 minutes. You should be looking to get your heart rate up to 60 to 70 per cent of its maximum, which you can do easily around a park or walking on the pavement.

- **LEVEL TWO:** If you go in here, then you need to step up your training to three to four times a week, going out for 30 minutes to an hour at a time. Your target zone for your heart rate should be 60 to 85 per cent of your maximum. You can get it up to this level by walking cross-terrain.

- **LEVEL THREE:** Go back to training three times a week and stay out for at least 40 minutes to an hour, keeping your heart rate working at 70 to 85 per cent of its maximum. You'll probably need to employ a few of the tricks mentioned in the Fat-burning section in order to keep your heart rate in the higher intensity zone.

# 6. Running

*Quicken your pace and reach your fitness goals more quickly*

There's no doubt about it, if you're coming to this programme with a reasonable standard of fitness and you're free from current or chronic injury, then running is a fantastic way to cut yourself into shape in the shortest time possible. The lads I had under my command during selection came to me in pretty

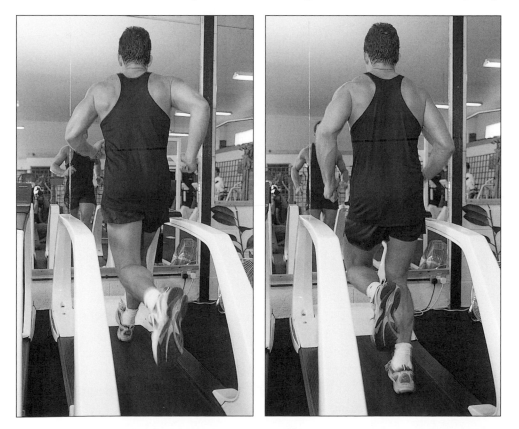

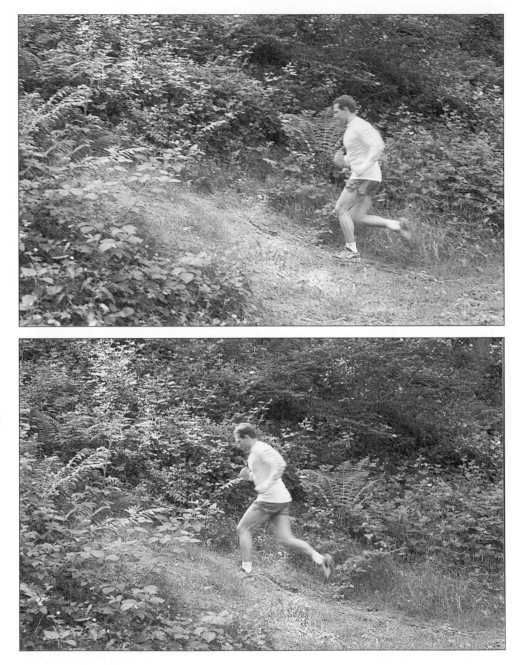

*I find running outdoors more beneficial than running on a machine because of the fresh air and the varied terrain.*

good condition, but that was nothing compared to how they ended up after a week doing runs of eight, 16 and 24 miles. They were super-fit in no time.

But the secret to a rewarding and injury-free running programme is to take it easy at first and slowly build the intensity and duration of your runs. There are a number of ways to do this, and I will cover them later in this section, but for now all you have to think about is how far and for how long you're going to start running. When people say they've just been for a run, unless they're wrapped in kitchen foil and have a gold medal, it usually means they've done two to three miles and have been out for about 20 to 40 minutes. That's not bad, but if you really want to start burning some weight off your body as well as increase your fitness you'll need to step that up to a minimum of 45 minutes. This is a great springboard for a successful running regime, and after a couple of weeks you should start to be able to push the time of your run up by 10 per cent every week.

When you start going a longer distance on the road try to pick up the pace over the last half-mile of a five-mile run; it's psychologically easier to do it towards the end when your personal finish line is in sight. Alternatively, you could throw in short, hard bursts throughout the run – by going up hills, for example, or by sprinting to a stop sign which is 50 yards ahead, easing off until your heart rate settles down, then taking off again for another landmark like a particular tree or lamp-post. This is good build-up for interval training, which you will progress to later.

The danger with running is that your body's joints have to absorb an enormous amount of shock every time your feet hit the ground, particularly if you're running on concrete. That's why it's very important that you warm up correctly. So before you get into the serious business of your run, jog lightly for ten minutes. Then, if you have time, stretch your quadriceps, hamstrings and calves. It's also essential that you stay hydrated throughout your run, so take on at least half a pint of water, half an hour before you begin, and try to have another half-pint for every 20 minutes you're on the road, then half a pint afterwards. Finally, don't forget to get rid of all that lactic acid which floods your muscles after you've been pushing them, with an efficient cool-down.

## Technique

There are two running phases: the impact phase and the flight phase. Impact is predictably when one foot is in contact with the ground, and flight is when both feet are in the air. Coaches are still undecided about the best way to let your foot hit the floor on a run. They aren't sure if runners should hit the ground with the ball of the foot first, or the heel. Olympic champions use both styles; what seems to separate them is the distance they run. Landing on the ball of the foot seems to be better suited to sprinters, whereas middle-distance runners use the middle of the foot and long-distance runners usually land from the heel to the toe. For biomechanical reasons you should adopt the latter technique.

Now here's a guide to how the rest of your body should shape up during a run.

- **UPPER BODY:** You should be leaning slightly forward as you run and, as with walking, the head should be held in a continuous line with your spine. To help you do this, think about looking forward so that your eyes meet the ground about 10 to 15 metres ahead of you.

- **ARMS:** Hold your arms close to your body at right angles to your elbow. Instead of swinging them parallel with your legs, you should think about swinging them at a slight angle, diagonally. Your left arm and right leg should move in the same direction at one time, and vice versa. Hold your hands in a loose fist, and don't let them rise above chest height on the upswing, or behind your hip bone on the backswing.

- **LEGS:** Your foot should hit the ground at the heel and then roll through the whole foot. If you can hear yourself running, i.e. you hear your feet slapping on the ground, then your technique is flawed. Your knees should be slightly flexed so that when your foot hits the ground your centre of gravity is lower, which stabilises your body throughout the motion. One of the keys to a successful technique is economy of effort, and this depends largely on your stride. Don't force your legs into an unnatural stride length, just go with what is most comfortable for you. Just remember that the longer the stride the more energy you're expending. Shorter strides are probably better when you're beginning because you'll run more economically, which means you'll run farther and do yourself more good.

- **BREATHING:** This can be difficult when you first start out as you will probably be out of breath, but don't gasp for air. Breathe evenly and naturally. Don't worry too much about your breathing, it tends to come automatically when you've got the other aspects of good technique squared away. When your technique is right you can think about adjusting your breathing rhythm to your running rhythm and getting the optimum oxygen exchange – which means that the emphasis should be on when you exhale, not inhale.

## Fat-burning

It's no accident that running is the most popular form of exercise among men because its weight-loss and fitness-boosting potential is immeasurable. For example, if you run at a steady 12-minute-mile pace you'll be burning roughly 10 calories a minute, and if you really step up the pace and start training with eight-minute miles, you'll burn 15 calories a minute. Interspersing a run with constant cool-downs is a great way to burn more fat, and is a stepping stone to interval training. For example, if you jog for five to eight minutes, then walk a minute, you'll burn 95 calories a mile; jogging continuously over this time period would only burn an extra five calories. To take your run to maximum efficiency, go for interval training. This means alternating periods of exercise during which you push yourself really hard with short periods of 'active rest', in which you lessen your effort but don't stop completely. The thing that you have to remember is that it's important to keep the ratio between going 'flat out' and your 'active rest' at one-to-one. You need to rest long enough to recover, but not so long that your heart rate drops to a level at which it's doing you little good. So aim to get your heart rate to 50 to 60 per cent of your heart-rate maximum for 'active rest', and then push on to 60 to 70 per cent of your heart-rate maximum when you decide to really go for it. This can be an effective fat-burner even when operated for a period as short as 20 to 30 minutes.

To give you some options, here are some other interval training examples:

- On a 30-minute run, go hard for two to four minutes, then go easy at a comfortable pace for the same length of time, then go hard again. Repeat the process until your 30 minutes is up.
- Run for four minutes (one-minute jog, two minutes hard run, one-minute jog), then walk for one minute. Now repeat these intervals eight times and you'll have benefited from the same training effect as you would have running eight times around a track.
- Run for nine minutes, then walk for one minute, then repeat these intervals 12 times. The effect is that of 120 minutes' endurance training without having weakened you body with a two-hour endurance run.

## Motivation

It can be pretty soul-destroying setting out on the same run time after time, even if you are interval training. So try a couple of the following strategies when it's starting to feel too much like hard work.

- Don't always run the same course in the same direction at the same time of day. Try and shake things up as much as you can, and if you run the same loop every day just run it in the opposite direction occasionally; you'll be amazed how this small variation totally changes your attitude and will make it feel like a completely different run.
- Run with mates. There's nothing better for motivation than a bit of competition, and this particularly applies with running.

- Go off-road. Running on pavements and roadsides can take its toll on your knees – and your lungs if you're running by a busy road. If you live in the country make use of the tracks and fields. If you live in the city then use the park.
- Don't be put off by the weather. As human beings we're always trying to talk ourselves out of things that we don't want to do and to make excuses for ourselves. It's either too cold, too wet or too dark to run. Make sure you've got the right equipment and you'll have one less excuse to let the weather interrupt your training.

## Training

- **LEVEL ONE:** Try to train four to five times a week. I know this sounds a lot, but at this level you don't have to be gone for hours, you're just trying to develop a solid base of fitness to build on. Your total running time for the week should be around one hour and you can break this up how you want – five 12-minute runs, three 20-minute runs and so on. This means that it's much easier to fit them in with your day. Don't go out for more than 30 minutes at a time during this level. Just make sure that you get your heart rate pumping at 50 to 60 per cent of its maximum for the majority of each run.

- **LEVEL TWO:** Bring your runs down to three per week and organise them so that your total running time for the week is two hours. Again, your training schedule can fit in with other demands on your time, so you can either go for two 45-minute runs and one 30-minute run, or four 30-minute runs. Just ensure that you don't go running for more than 45 minutes at a time, and that your heart rate is working between 60 and 70 per cent of its maximum when you're out. When you feel that you've got enough energy to carry on for longer than 45 minutes, you should think about stepping up to level three.

- **LEVEL THREE:** Step your total running time up to three hours a week and try to get out between three and six times a week. Split it up with three 60-minute runs, four 45-minute runs, five 35-minute runs, and so on. Make sure that your minimum run is 35 minutes long and your maximum 70 minutes, and try to get your maximum heart rate in the 70 to 80 per cent zone for some of that time, perhaps with interval training.

# 7. Cycling

## *A performance exercise that will separate you from the chasing pack*

Whether it's a mountain bike, your old racer or an exercise bike, cycling has the advantage of being a low-impact aerobic drill that can facilitate fitness in double-quick time. So if you're coming back from injury or have weak joints, then cycling is the first performance exercise that you should think about using to get you fit. Whether you're cycling outdoors or on a stationary bike, the key is to aim occasionally for a pace that's a little uncomfortable – because effective calorie-burning is always going to be dependent on the speed or intensity you're maintaining. And the great thing with a bike is that there are a ton of easy ways to introduce this intensity into your workout, whether it's a hill on a racing bike, rough terrain on a mountain bike, or a higher resistance setting on a stationary bike.

Cycling outside offers instant motivation because it's seen as more of a 'fun' activity than either walking or running. Cycling through mountainous terrain or countryside instantly takes your mind off the fact that you're actually working hard and getting fit. This is why more people stick to a cycling

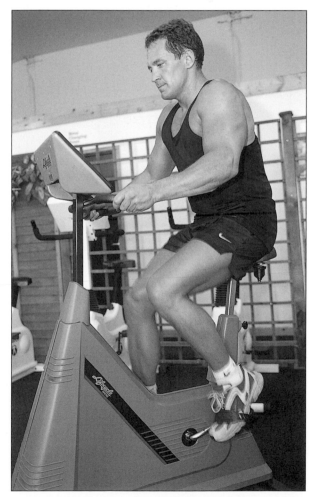

training programme than many of the other aerobic drills that are perceived to be harder work. The downside of this is that cycling through pleasant surroundings can distract you from the task in hand and you can all too easily begin to cruise through your time on the road without really doing yourself any good.

This is where mountain biking has the edge over road work: when you go off road and on to tracks it's not often that you'll find yourself at the kind of steady cruise that you might fall into on a long, straight road. Traditional cycling puts all the emphasis on your legs, but when you're off road your upper body also has a lot of work to do in order to keep your body and the bike in balance. It's this difference that makes mountain biking the most complete cycling drill you can do as the varied terrain forces you to use a lot more energy.

When it comes to using a stationary cycle at home or in the gym, you are dependent on the resistance lever to construct your own imaginary terrain and simulate the fitness benefits of cycling outside. The main advantage of a stationary cycle is that you never have to worry about your training being interrupted by heavy traffic or slowed down by a particularly tricky bit of terrain.

## Technique

Whatever kind of bike you have, you need to ensure that it's set up correctly according to your height and frame. So make sure you've got the saddle at the right height before you set off anywhere. You should find that when you're cycling and each foot hits the bottom of its pedalling arc that your knee is slightly flexed by about 10 to 15 degrees. Another test is to see if your body rocks from side to side when you pedal, if it does then your seat is too high. To sort out any problems sit on your bike and lean on a wall to hold yourself steady while you bring both pedals up to the horizontal position. When your knee is exactly vertical above the axle of the front pedal with both the balls of your feet on the pedals, the seat is in its best position.

- **UPPER BODY:** As long as you're not thinking about going after a yellow jersey any time soon, you don't have to worry about adopting the kind of static, aerodynamic posture you'll see from professional cyclists. This is unnatural for most off-road biking anyway, and you should be doing the opposite throughout your ride, changing your grip and seating position as often as possible so as to prevent muscles cramping and to reduce any strain on your joints.

- **ARMS:** Just make sure that you're able to reach the handlebars by leaning forward slightly with your back straight. Keep your elbows bent so that you're riding in the most aerodynamic position without taking it to extremes and hunching down over your handlebars.

- **LEGS:** Most cyclists simply push the pedal down and let the bike mechanism bring it up around again, but there's a lot more to pedalling than this. What you want to do is work the pedal around in the biggest arc possible, pushing down as you lower it and pulling it up as far as you can to the rear; to do this you'll need pedal straps. When you're doing it right, your foot will alternate between pointing up and down during one revolution of the pedal; your foot should never be flat throughout the entire revolution. Admittedly, the faster you go the more difficult this will become, and sometimes you won't be able to help your feet staying almost flat throughout one revolution. However, whenever you can you should make sure that you are pedalling, so as to give your legs maximum benefit. Stand and pedal for 15 to 20 seconds after 15 minutes in the saddle to relieve saddle pressure and stop your muscles cramping.

- **BREATHING:** Just try to breathe naturally, which will become easier as your technique becomes more solid.

## Fat-burning

The one problem with cycling in terms of fat-burning is that your training can be held up easily. That's why you want to ensure that wherever you train you're going to be able to work as hard as you want, whenever you want. This is one of the advantages of a stationary bike, in that it guarantees you'll be able to stay in your target heart-rate zone for the length of time you want. So if you're finding it hard to cycle outdoors and stick to the training plan below, switch to a stationary cycle. If you don't have access to one you should think about buying a 'turbo trainer' from your local bike shop, which effectively jacks up the back wheel of your normal bike and allows you to pedal your heart out without actually going anywhere. If you belong to a gym you should try a spinning programme, which usually involves joining in a group session headed by a coach. The programme simulates cycling outdoors by varying speed, riding position and resistance.

If you're determined to train in the fresh air, try doing a couple of hill intervals. All you have to do is find a hill or incline in your locality, bordered by some flat surface. After you've warmed up sufficiently on the flat ground start your intervals up the hill. Begin by taking it easy for three minutes, then ride all out for three; go back to riding easy for five minutes, then ride hard for five; slow it down for three minutes, then go all out again for three, continuing like this until you run out of hill. Cool down with an easy ride back down the hill. If the hill is quite short, just repeat the process until you've fulfilled your training requirements. The beauty of it is that – because the whole thing takes place on a gradient – you're forced to recover while you're still climbing which means you've got no choice but to keep your heart rate at a productive level throughout.

## Motivation

As I've already discussed it's all too easy to reach a kind of hypnotic state when cycling outside, and to end up cruising through your drill without paying too much attention to what your heart-rate is doing. A great way to make sure this doesn't happen is to get together with some mates and cycle in an interval pace line (as you often see in Olympic events), riding single file and tightly packed, about three feet from each other. You should start out at the front and, after warming up for a while, step up into a higher gear and increase the pace for two minutes. This is really hard work and should get your heart rate right up as you make a slipstream for the riders behind you. After your time is up, break away and drop to the back of the line, where you will be able to enjoy riding in someone else's slipstream. Drop down to a lower gear and cycle faster so that your heart rate maintains the right intensity, and you stay in your target zone. You always need to be thinking about pedalling faster rather than harder. Spinning in a low gear is the way to do this (the most efficient pedalling range is 80 to 100 revolutions per minute). This process will continue with riders pulling from the front then breaking off and dropping back until you find yourself at the front of the line again. You can keep training like this for as long as you want.

## Training

- **LEVEL ONE:** Try to train two to three times a week and stay out for anything between 15 minutes and 45 minutes. Warm up until your heart rate has reached between 60 and 70 per cent of its maximum, then stay in this zone for anything between 10 minutes and 35 minutes. If it's possible for you to ride to work (and the ride is long enough), then this is a great level to combine training with your daily schedule.

- **LEVEL TWO:** Make sure you have got enough time to get out there three times a week, and build up the length of your ride so that you're cycling each time for an hour. After your warm-up you should be aiming to get your heart rate working at 60 to 75 per cent of its maximum for as much of the ride as possible.

- **LEVEL THREE:** You should be looking to push up your maximum heart-rate percentage to the 70 to 85 per cent region for a significant amount of time during your ride, e.g. 40 minutes of a 60-minute ride, or 60 minutes of a 100-minute ride.

# 8. Swimming

## *For a great physique and fitness to match, just add water*

Swimming is up there with cycling when it comes to finding a low-impact aerobic drill that offers a head-to-toe workout. This is because the buoyancy of the water supports the whole body while providing an environment of natural resistance that increases your energy expenditure with every movement, calling into action almost every major muscle group in the body. And because you'll be calling upon muscles that you didn't even know you had, it's essential that you warm up first. You should try to swim 100 metres crawl, then switch to backstroke for 50 metres, and finish off with 50 metres of breaststroke for your warm-up. As you get more familiar with the activity, step this up to 200 metres of crawl and 100 metres of backstroke and breaststroke before you get into the main body of your training.

Similarly, when you've finished training you should wait a few minutes before you leave the pool and cool down, spending your time on a light backstroke or breaststroke while you wait for your heartbeat to return to normal.

Your swimming training won't be so dependent on heart-rate maximums because of certain problems caused by wearing the transmitter in a water environment. Pool water with a high chlorine content can be conductive and the electrodes of the transmitter can be short-circuited. Also, the extreme body movement that is natural with swimming strokes can shift the transmitter to a point where it's no longer possible to pick up the ECG signal.

This is why the best way to set out your training is with intervals – i.e. a number of swims (sets) split up by bouts of rest (interval). However, unlike the other aerobic drills where your intervals compose 'active' rest, with swimming you want to just hang on to the wall after you've given your all and prepare yourself for the next bout of heavy swimming. So you could do 10 50-metre crawls, with a one-minute interval between each; or five 100-metre crawls with a two-minute interval.

Whatever stroke you're doing, you need to concentrate on the two phases that make up one revolution: propulsion and relaxation. The propulsion phase is when your arms are forcing a volume of water behind you to propel you forward, while relaxation is usually when your hands are out of the water and aren't experiencing any resistance. In order to keep going for the lengths of time set out in the training programme you need to be able to introduce your muscle fibres to brief periods of rest during the stroke revolutions. So when you feel your limbs becoming tired you should focus on lengthening the relaxation phase a little longer, i.e. extending the phase in the breaststroke.

## Technique

Swimming is unlike all the other aerobic drills in that, unless you're a webbed-wonder, it's going to take you some time to get your technique right. All the standard strokes – front crawl, backstroke, breaststroke and butterfly – are more technical than any of the other drills in the book, so be patient and expect a good degree of coughing and spluttering at the side of the pool before you make great advances with your training.

However, all the strokes can be achieved with some practice, and once you hone your technique to a reasonable level the rewards will be well worth it.

The key to an efficient swimming technique, no matter what stroke you are using, is 'hydrostatic lift'. The classic demonstration of hydrostatic lift is to lie on your back in the water and lift your arms and legs out of the water; you will find that your torso is sucked down. What this demonstrates is that the more of your body you keep submerged, the more buoyant you are, and you will need less force to cut you through the water, so your stroke becomes more efficient. For example, when you're doing the crawl you should try to keep your head as far under the water as you can at all times. On the subject of keeping your head under water, it's important that you remember to keep your eyes open – nothing will sink a swimming programme faster than careering into someone while you're going full speed ahead. If you're not aware of your surroundings it's all too easy to lose your sense of direction and drift out of your lane and into someone else's. If your eyes are particularly sensitive to chlorinated water, purchase a pair of goggles.

### FRONT CRAWL

- **UPPER BODY:** Your upper body will roll to either side to allow alternate hands to reach in front of it and grab a volume of water.

- **ARMS:** The propulsion phase begins as you force a volume of water behind you with your hand and arm. Your hand should be shaped in a paddle with your fingers closed, and your arm will trace a key-shaped pattern through the water. By the time your hand and arm come level with your shoulder under the water, your upper arm should be at 90-degrees to your shoulder under your body, with the elbow bent so that you present the maximum amount of surface area for the water to react against. The final stage of the propulsion phase is complete when the arm extends to the side of the body. For the relaxation stage the hand and arm come out of the water to reach forward, close to the body, before dropping back into the water when the revolution starts again.

- **LEGS:** Your legs should be kicking to assist in taking you forward and to keep your body stabilised as it rolls from side to side. Don't just kick from the knee joint – the kick should come from the hip, which pushes the upper leg downwards. This one action against the resistance of the water will automatically produce the required effect for the rest of your leg. Your feet should point slightly inward and there should be three leg kicks for each stage of the arm movement.

- **BREATHING:** You should be exhaling throughout the propulsion stage, as your arm comes back under your body. Inhale on the relaxation phase, when your body rolls to allow your other hand to reach for the next volume of water.

## BACKSTROKE

- **UPPER BODY:** Your body should automatically roll to the side of the arm cutting through the water.

- **ARMS:** Make sure on the relaxation phase (as each arm is brought into the pool) that you cut the water with your little finger first. On the propulsion phase the arm should push forward and down a little. Your hand and arm should now begin forcing the water back, and as your arm comes level with your shoulder your hand, elbow and shoulder should form a vertical triangle; after this stage your hand and arm move to your upper leg. As your hand surfaces again on the relaxation phase it should cut the water with the index finger first; your arm should be extended and should move parallel to the body.

- **LEGS:** Your legs should be kicking to assist your arm movement in propelling you forward and to keep your body stabilised as it rolls from side to side. As with the front crawl, don't just kick from the knee joint but from the hip. You should have completed six kicks for one revolution of your arm.

- **BREATHING:** You should be inhaling while the arm is windmilling over your head and down into the water (the relaxation phase); and exhaling on the propulsion phase as your arm moves under the water.

## BREASTSTROKE

- **UPPER BODY:** Bad technique in this stroke can place undue strain on the neck and lower back, so it's important that you get it right. Begin by relaxing your upper body and not struggling to keep your head above water all the time. Instead, you should be looking towards the bottom of the pool as you propel yourself forward with only the top of your head above water. This goes back to the principle of hydrostatic lift: the more of your body you keep submerged the more buoyant you are, making the stroke more efficient. Your head and shoulders will only clear the water at the end of the propulsion stage.

- **ARMS:** As you push off for your first stroke your head will be under the water and your arms will be extended in front of your face, palms facing outwards and knuckles facing each other a few inches apart. Each hand and arm should separate a volume of water and drag it back behind you to propel yourself forwards, your palms facing away from your body with your fingers together. Once your hands are in line with your shoulders you should pull them together quickly and stretch them out ahead of your face, which will again be looking down at the bottom of the pool.

- **LEGS:** As your arms are brought back during the propulsion stage you should initiate a 'frog kick', whereby your feet are brought towards your rear with your knees bent, then kicked in a semicircular movement. The leg movement ends by closing the legs quickly when they're almost fully extended, the soles of your feet pointing inwards.

- **BREATHING:** When your head and shoulders clear the water at their highest point during the gliding or relaxation stage you should be inhaling. During the propulsion, when you are under water, you should exhale.

## BUTTERFLY

- **UPPER BODY:** This is the most difficult stroke to master, because your body has to zigzag through the water in a movement initiated by the head and upper body. Your head should come out of the water during the propulsion stage, and during the relaxation stage your head should hit the water before your arms and hands.

- **ARMS:** They should move simultaneously with synchronisation as they come forward and downward into the water. Turn your hands slightly outwards when your hands reach your shoulders and cut the water with all your fingers. Under the water your arms should trace a key-shaped trail (as with the front crawl), the hands meeting beneath the chest and pushing away towards the upper legs.

- **LEGS:** During one revolution of your arms you should have kicked twice, the first coming as your arms enter the water and the second as your arms propel you forward. As with the crawl, the movement should start from the hip, the difference here being that your legs stay together throughout and operate the kick as one. In this way there is a wave movement produced. Keep your feet relaxed and turned inwards slightly during the downward phase of the kick.

- **BREATHING:** Inhale during the propulsion phase, as your arms and head emerge from the water, exhale as you drop down into the water again.

## Fat-burning

Swimming has been much maligned as an aerobic drill because it's thought that you can't burn fat effectively. This is true if your idea of a swim is a couple of dive-bombs in the deep end and then half a width, but if you swap the dive-bombs for a front crawl and the widths for lengths then you can end up burning around 540 calories per hour. If you're looking to get the maximum amount of burn in the minimum amount of time then you need to think about reducing the time of your interval. Keeping the interval between sets at around 15 to 40 seconds will see you make radical fitness gains, because it will keep your heart rate pumping at around 60 to 85 per cent of its maximum. If you're doing a number of short swims in a set (e.g. five 100-metre swims) rest for only about 15 seconds between each; for longer swims allow up to 40 seconds for recovery.

## Motivation

It is easy to get disillusioned with swimming because of the highly technical nature of the exercise. So don't asume that the techniques outlined are written in stone; far from it, you should use the guidelines to develop a stroke that is efficient and fast for you. Mix your speeds and strokes to avoid falling into a stale routine, where you swim the same distance with the same stroke during every training session. Occasionally, speed up your lengths as well, because the faster you swim the harder your muscles and your heart will work. If you decide to introduce sprint sets into your training, do it early on while your muscles are able to sustain the effort. This will also mean that you'll have to rest for longer to maximise your energy expenditure during the sets.

## *Training*

- **LEVEL ONE:** Try to train three times a week, and do five 100 metres of front crawl, resting for 15-second intervals. When you can do this and retain more energy, rest for two to three minutes and complete the intervals in level two as well.

- **LEVEL TWO:** Train three to four times a week. Each set consists of doing 200 metres of front crawl, then 100 metres of either backstroke or breaststroke. Do this six times, resting for intervals of 40 seconds. When you can complete the intervals in level one and two, rest for two to three minutes and do all the intervals in level three.

- **LEVEL THREE:** Try to train three times a week, swimming all four strokes within a set. The first sprint should be butterfly, then backstroke, then breaststroke, then front crawl. If you haven't mastered butterfly then substitute a front crawl. Do twelve 25-metre sprints with an interval of 15 seconds in between each sprint. Rest for two to three minutes before you go into the next set.

# 9. Indoor rowing

## *Going nowhere fast can be a great way to get fit*

The rise of the rowing machine means that an effective aerobic drill that was pretty inaccessible before has now become widely available; and you don't even have to get your feet wet. In fact, the rowing machine can provide an

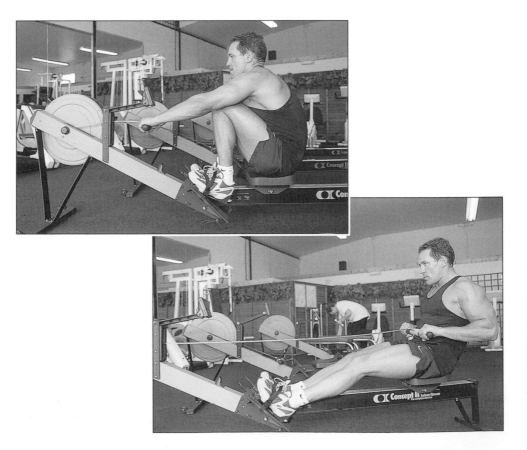

even better workout than the real thing, because the flywheel mechanism (or ergometer) doesn't assist you in any way at all (unlike a boat), and so guarantees maximum energy output.

Like swimming and cycling, this is a weight-bearing exercise that offers total body conditioning. However, rowing differs in that the machine also supplies you with a wealth of electronic data that you can use to fine-tune your training and keep it efficient. If you walk into any gym it's likely that you'll find a machine made by Concept II, complete with a performance monitor that, most importantly, provides an interface for a heart-rate monitor. This automatically picks up the ECG data from your chest belt and displays it on the screen in front of you as you row, allowing you to keep both hands busy and track your heart's output. The monitor also provides a lot of other information that can help you shape your workout: as well as your elapsed time or metres, your stroke rate, total output, and output for each stroke per 500 metres. All this data allows you to work with pyramids, intervals or by your heart rate.

## Technique

Although not as difficult technically as rowing on a river – because you don't have to contend with external factors like choppy water or direction changes – the technique on a rowing machine still consists of the three basic movements of catch, drive and finish. The catch comes as you slide the seat forward, the drive as you power back with the legs and upper body, and the finish as you pull the handle into your mid-section. Perfecting each phase will leave you with an efficient technique that couples a relaxed grip on the handle with a powerful driving motion that begins from the legs, then transfers to the rest of the body and through the machine itself.

- **UPPER BODY:** Relax your shoulders and brace your back in the upright position. At the finish, don't pull the handle up too high. This will cause you to lean back too far and put your back in a weak position. You should be drawing the handle into the midriff. Never start the drive (or try to get more leverage) by pulling back with the upper body, as this can lead to injury. Instead, start the drive with the legs and lever the body back with straight arms, ready to take up the drive by transferring the power of your legs into the stroke through your arms and on to the handle.

- **ARMS:** As you draw the handle into your body, your wrists and forearms should be horizontal, and your elbows should finish up past your body.

During the catch phase you need to keep in mind the sequence: hands, body, slide. This should help you to remember that only after your arms have fully extended and your body has come forward should you slide forward, maintaining the arm and body position – you should never be sliding forward before the handle has gone past your knees. If your hands hit your knees or you have to lift the handle in order to clear your knees, then you know your technique isn't quite right. Remember that your arms should be fully extended and relaxed during the catch.

*Try and vary your training. Canoeing down a river can be more fun than doing the exercises on a machine.*

- **LEGS:** Always start the drive by pushing with the legs, but don't push away too early because the back won't be braced and the power won't be transferred onto the handle.

- **BREATHING:** Inhale on the catch and exhale on the drive.

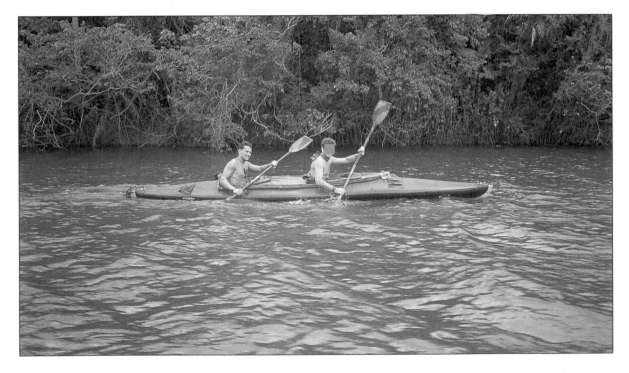

## Fat-burning

You'll burn 500 to 700 calories per hour when you're rowing at the intensities detailed in the training section. It's important not to be misled into thinking that the higher you set the resistance on the ergometer the more fat you will fry during your workout. I still see loads of guys flick the ergometer to 10 and then really go for it, but they're knackered after 10 minutes. When you're on a rower you're not interested in creating a high force to work against – that's what weightlifting circuits are for. It's not about the resistance you're rowing against, but the length of time that you stay on the rower at the required heart-rate level. You don't want the length and quality of your training to be limited by muscular fatigue before your body has had a chance to benefit. So aim for a setting with which you can achieve your training goal, usually around the six or seven mark.

## Motivation

Use the performance monitor to mix up your training. For example, if you feel you need a change from the heart-rate programme, then you can try working pyramid or interval sessions. What follows is an example of a reverse pyramid session. You begin by rowing for a certain length of time at a certain pace, then reduce the time and pace in increments until you reach a base level, at which you start to build back up until you end up where you started. You can increase the time of the pyramid session as much as you want; just make sure that the final level always corresponds with the first.

- Row four minutes at a pace of 2 mins 20 secs per 500m.
- Row three minutes at a pace of 2 mins 15 secs per 500m.
- Row two minutes at a pace of 2 mins 10 secs per 500m.
- Row one minute at a pace of 2 mins 5 secs per 500m.
- Row two minutes at a pace of 2 mins 10 secs per 500m.
- Row three minutes at a pace of 2 mins 15 secs per 500m.
- Row four minutes at a pace of 2 mins 20 secs per 500m.

Interval training on a rowing machine is similar to the other drills that employ 'active rest' whereby you work hard for an interval, slow it down for an interval, then repeat the process. In this way you can maintain your heart rate at a positive intensity for longer, and this has an excellent effect on your overall conditioning. When this gets too easy you can increase the intervals during which you're rowing hard, so that you're rowing for 45, 60 or 90 seconds. Make sure this corresponds with an increase in the pace at which you're rowing. The following table is an example of an interval session.

- Row five minutes at a pace of about 2 mins 15 secs per 500m.
- Row hard for 30 seconds at a pace of about 1 min 55 secs per 500m.
- Row one minute at a pace of about 2 mins 25 secs per 500m.
- Now repeat the last two intervals six times.

# *Training*

- **LEVEL ONE:** Try to train three times a week. In your first session go easy, with 10 to 15 minutes at 65 per cent of your maximum heart rate. For your next two sessions row for 20 minutes at 70 to 75 per cent, and for your final session stay on for 30 minutes, pushing your heart rate up to 75 per cent of its maximum.

- **LEVEL TWO:** Try to maintain 65 per cent for 30 to 40 minutes in your first weekly session. Increase this to 70 per cent for 30 to 40 minutes for session two, and 70 per cent for 30 to 50 minutes for your final weekly session.

- **LEVEL THREE:** Increase the number of times you train to four times a week. Maintain 65 per cent of your maximum heart rate, and increase the length of time that you're on the rower for each session by the following:
  - session one, 30 to 50 minutes
  - session two, 40 to 60 minutes
  - session three, 40 to 70 minutes
  - session four, 40 to 80 minutes

# 10. Weight training

*Your body's been on stand-by for too long.
Here's how to kick it into action with weights,
and get results fast*

It's no joke that having extra muscle saved my life. If I hadn't just finished with the counter-terrorist (special projects) team before going into Iraq I probably wouldn't have come back from the Gulf. Because of special projects I was physically the strongest I had ever been and had built up a lot of muscle on my upper body. Not only had I been hitting the weights hard, but a lot of extra strength had come from the unusual body work I had been doing – going up or sliding down ropes, climbing into buildings, carrying guys, jumping off vehicles, pushing people away or restraining them. On top of all this, I was handling a lot of weight: body armour, Kevlar helmet and waistcoat loaded with ammunition, stun-grenades and axes, as well as my machine-gun and pistol. Obviously, this isn't something you will have to worry about, but committing yourself to the weight circuits on the following pages will reward you with the same kind of strength gains I experienced. Of course, your current level of fitness will dictate where you begin, so be realistic. If the most exercise you've had

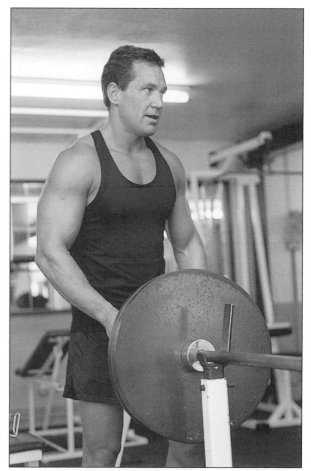

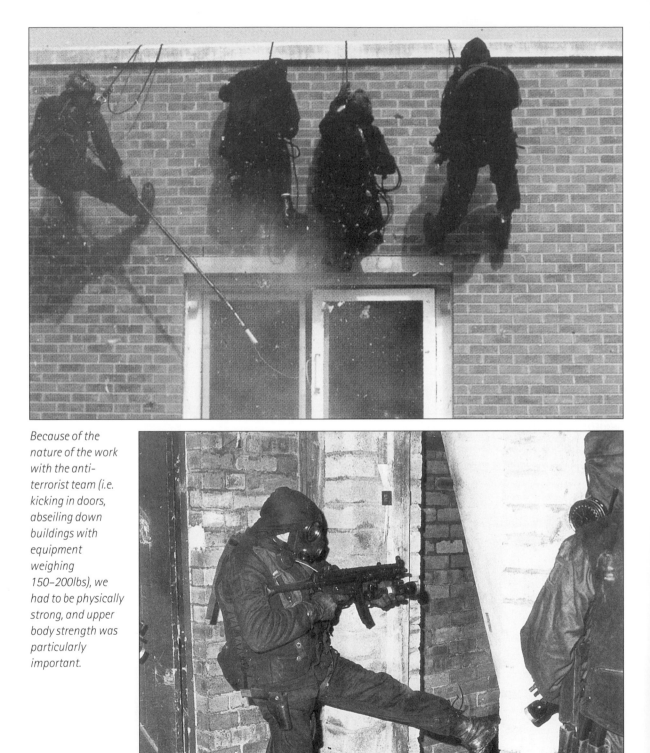

*Because of the nature of the work with the anti-terrorist team (i.e. kicking in doors, abseiling down buildings with equipment weighing 150–200lbs), we had to be physically strong, and upper body strength was particularly important.*

recently is disposing of the rubbish left over from last night's curry, then don't kid yourself that you can go straight to level three. Not only will it be too much for you, it will probably put you off for life and injure you in the process. (If it makes you feel any better, I've had to put my time in at level one as well, especially when I was recuperating after my escape from Iraq.)

So here's a final briefing that will hopefully clear up any questions you have about strength training in general and performing the circuits, leaving you free to take care of business on the weight bench.

## WHICH IS BETTER – FREE WEIGHTS OR MACHINES?

They tend to complement one another and make for a more complete work-out – which is why I use a mixture of both in my programme. Free weights bring the maximum number of muscles into play during a single exercise, because they tend to involve timing and balance as well as strength. Machines reduce the need for the first two qualities, as their mechanisms do most of the work for you. However, when you're on a machine you know that your form is less likely to suffer and the targeted muscles are really being put under pressure.

There's always a free-weight equivalent for a machine exercise, so if you're having difficulty getting access to a particular machine do the free-weight version.

## HOW OFTEN SHOULD I TRAIN?

People often ask me how much weight training they need to do to see significant strength gains and reach the point where their bodies are constantly ticking over and burning excess fat. With my programme you can achieve substantial results at level one by training just three days a week. But the more effort you put into the programme, the more you'll get out of it. So once you progress to the other levels – or if you're fit enough to go in at a higher level from the outset – you'll need to work a split circuit and train four to six times a week. Just to give you an indication of what each level entails, I've broken them down for you.

- **LEVEL ONE – THE START-UP CIRCUIT:** This means working out three times a week and is your starting point if you've been leading a pretty inactive lifestyle for some time, have been out of action for a shorter while, or just want to lose fat and tone your muscles without increasing their size. You'll hit each of the major muscle groups (chest, back, shoulders, legs, biceps, triceps and abdominals) with the most basic exercises to build up a solid foundation of strength. Move up to the next level when you find

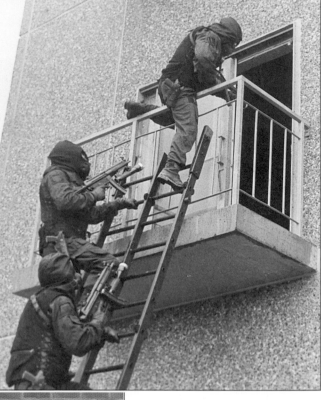

*Running up a ladder to enter a building. This is where quality aerobic training and strong legs come into play.*

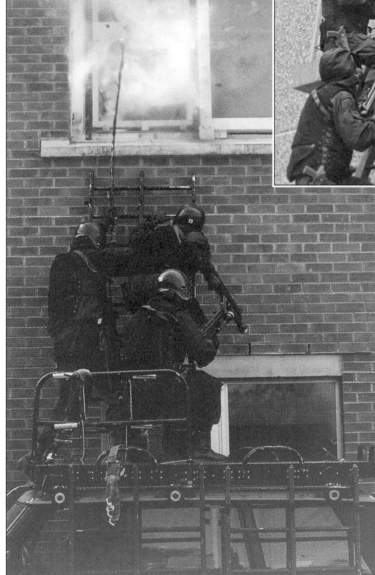

that you aren't making any more significant strength gains or that you're plateauing (see Dangers and Setbacks, page 13). If your goal is purely fat reduction, stick at this level while you do your aerobic drills but up the repetitions, i.e. instead of doing three sets of 12, do three sets of 20 which will burn your fat and tone your muscles. Remember that your muscles will feel sore for the first couple of weeks after starting training – this is normal and a good sign that you're targeting the right muscles.

- **LEVEL TWO – THE SPLIT-CIRCUITS:** When you go in at this level you still need to be prepared to work out three times a week, but you'll pick up the intensity – increasing the number of sets and weight, but lowering the repetitions. You'll begin to hit each body part with a number of exercises instead of just the one. How you split the routine is up to you and your schedule, but ideally you'll be working out Monday, Wednesday and Friday.

    You can continue with these circuits for as long as you're happy with the benefits that you're getting from them. But when you start cruising through the circuits or you stop seeing results in the mirror you should start mixing things up. When you fail to see any strength gains with this kind of workout it's time to move up to level three.

- **LEVEL THREE – THE ADVANCED SPLIT CIRCUITS:** When I'm at my peak this is my personal routine. You should bring these circuits into play when any of your level-two workouts become unproductive, and be prepared to work four days on, one day off. It's essential that you have a rest day because this routine is intensive. You'll train the chest and biceps on day one; shoulders on day two; legs on day three; and back and triceps on day four. The fifth day will be a rest day, then you'll begin the process again. You'll really start packing on the weight here but you'll be doing four to five sets, starting off with one set of 12 reps (which really acts as a warm-up using light weights). By the time you get down to the fifth set, you'll just be doing a couple of reps with a heavy weight and a spotter, which is what really builds your strength. On the rest day you'll still go for your walk or do your chosen aerobic drill. The advanced split circuits are designed to stop your workout from plateauing (see Dangers and Setbacks, page 13) and hit all the muscle groups hard. You're now training as hard as an SAS soldier.

## WHAT ABOUT GETTING A SIX-PACK?

There are lots of abdominal exercises, but I have selected the ones that work best for me. My abdominal work consists of four exercises: crunches,

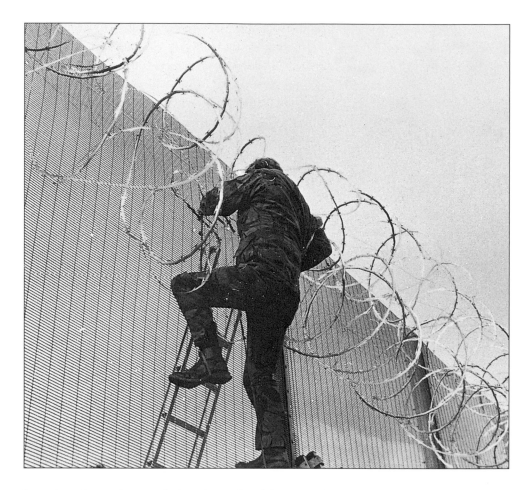

*A lot of SAS guys would rather go AWOL than face the level-three workout!*

hanging-leg raises, side bends and cable crunches. I do them on every work-out day and will use them as a warm-up and a break between training specific body parts in the workouts. I rely on high repetitions to failure without using any weight (except on side bends where I use a very light dumb-bell). I don't use any weight because you don't want to build any thickness around your waist – the aim is to keep it as narrow and trim as possible.

Diet and nutrition is essential for achieving a six-pack, because you may have the best defined six-pack in the world, but if there's a layer of fat covering it you're not going to see it. Don't kid yourself that you can burn fat solely from your belly by doing sit-ups (known as spot reducing) – losing weight is a whole body process.

## WHICH AREAS OF MY BODY SHOULD I TRAIN?

Your arms, shoulders, chest, back, stomach, legs and abdominals – I've made sure that all these areas are targeted in the circuits. You tend to find that the smaller muscles in your body get worked as a consequence of working the larger areas – for example, your forearm muscles will be in constant use as you grip and use the weights, and will still get worked even though you're not targeting them directly.

## HOW MUCH SHOULD I BE LIFTING?

The weight you lift will vary according to the strength that you bring to the programme, but ultimately you need to be expending 65 to 70 per cent of your energy per set. This means starting with a weight that you will struggle to lift on the last repetition of a set, but not so much that it's going to knacker you or restrict you from doing more sets. This is going to mean a little trial and error to begin with, so always start light so you're never in danger of damaging yourself. If you find the weight is too light for you, increase it on the next set.

The important thing is not to get sucked into looking at what other people are pushing in the gym, because this is where you can get yourself injured with torn muscles that put you out of the game before you've begun. The fact that someone may be pushing 180kg on the bench press on the other side of the gym and you can hardly lift the bar doesn't mean a thing. You are feeling the same resistance that he's feeling, so go in and experiment with weight and build gradually.

For a lot of the exercises, I suggest that to develop and avoid plateauing you should increase the weight by about 1.1kg to 2.3kg each week. This is called double-progressive training. For example, if you can manage eight repetitions on the close-grip bench press (the first exercise in level one), with around 22kg on the bar, then keep training until you can do the maximum repetitions that I suggest for that exercise – in this case 10. Then increase the weight by 1.1kg. You'll probably only be able to do eight repetitions before failure, but keep training until you can manage 10, then increase the weight again until you've got an extra 2.2kg on the bar. Again, you'll probably go down to eight repetitions but can work back up to 10 repetitions. You can repeat this process for a while before you'll probably plateau, which is when you can employ some other tricks or step up to the next level and do different exercises.

## HOW MUCH TIME SHOULD I LEAVE
## FOR MY MUSCLES TO RECOVER?

After you've finished a set your muscles always need time to recover before you can call upon them to perform again. You need at least a couple of minutes between sets to give your nervous system a chance to regain its lifting capabilities. When I get back into training after a lay-off, starting at level one, I'll allow myself between 90 and 120 seconds' rest between each set. At level two I'll start thinking about cutting down my recovery time to about 75 seconds so that when I reach level three I'm giving myself exactly one minute's rest between each set. As for the time between the circuits themselves, you need to allow 24 to 48 hours to rest your muscles' fibres and allow them to recharge and rebuild. This is why the split circuits are so effective – because you can work one body part on one day and then allow it to rest for a day or two while you work on another.

## HOW LONG SHOULD I STAY AT MY CHOSEN LEVEL?

When you notice that you've stopped making strength gains or you've stopped seeing any differences in your body shape, you're probably plateauing (see Dangers and Setbacks, page 13), so to kick-start your workout go to the next level.

## WILL LIFTING WEIGHTS HELP ME LOSE WEIGHT?

Absolutely. The strength gains you will experience from the circuits and the corresponding increase in muscle mass on your body has a knock-on effect that helps you keep excess weight off your frame. It's a fact that lifting weights in conjunction with a cutback in calorie-intake will burn up more fat

*This is what happens when you have a great Christmas and New Year! Following the steps in my programme, you can achieve improved fitness and physique, as well as significant weight loss.*

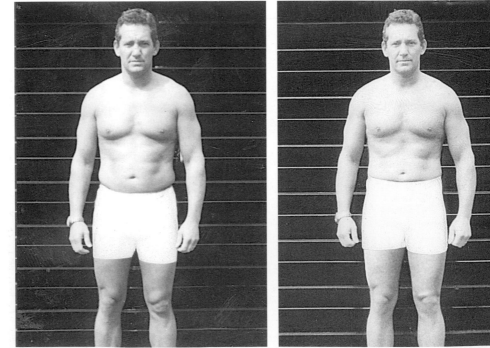

Week 1

Week 2

and less muscle tissue. Your body becomes a metabolic machine because muscle tissue burns more calories than fat tissue even when you're resting – so it's a win-win situation.

## HOW LONG WILL IT TAKE UNTIL I START SEEING A DIFFERENCE?

Don't expect any significant changes for a month. I know that sounds harsh, but it's the truth – and there's no point in me telling you that it's going to happen any sooner.

A great motivational tool to get through this first month is to take a photo of yourself when you begin the training and put it away in a drawer. Take another one a month later and compare the two. You'll be amazed at the difference (regardless of the condition you were in to begin with, because the changes are all relative). Look at the pictures on this page of the last time I began the training programme. These were taken over a period of four to six weeks, and although I felt that I didn't look any different from when I started, you can clearly see that my body was changing. This is because you see yourself every day and don't notice the gradual change in physique – but seeing the results of your circuits and drills dramatically displayed like this makes you want to train even more.

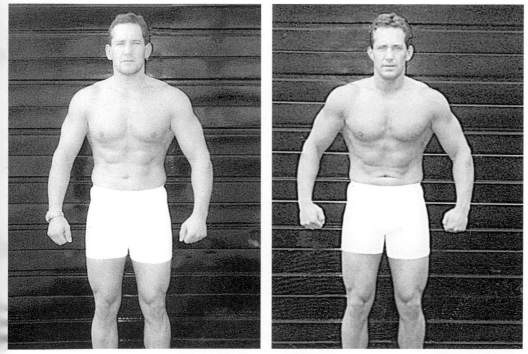

*Week 4*                    *Week 6*

# 11. The exercises

## i) Chest

### BENCH PRESS

Lie on the weight bench with your head under the bar-bell rack and your feet flat on the floor. Your thumbs should be roughly over your shoulders. Make sure your hands are far enough apart to let your forearm form a right angle with your upper arm at the bottom of the movement (practise with an imaginary bar-bell). Your wrists should be firm, with your palms facing your feet as you grip the bar. Now lift the bar-bell off the rack and lock it above your chest at arm's length. Slowly bend your elbows, lowering the weight to the middle of your chest. It should touch it gently, more or less in the centre of your breastbone. Hold for a second, then slowly press the bar-bell back up to the starting position.

**FORM GUIDE:** As you lift the weight think about moving the bar in a shallow J-shape to focus the exercise on the targeted muscles. If you push it straight up and down you'll be lowering the bar to your throat, which puts a lot of strain on your shoulders.

Once you start pressing heavier weights you need to make sure you've got a spotter helping you to lift and lower the bar (see Figure 1). You'll know when you're lifting too much weight because your feet will come off the floor and your back will begin to arch – this puts a lot of pressure on your spine and can lead to injury (see Figure 2).

**MUSCLES TARGETED:** Pectoral, tricep, deltoid.

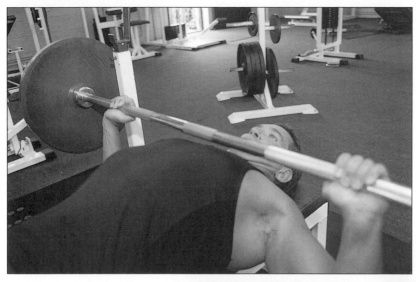

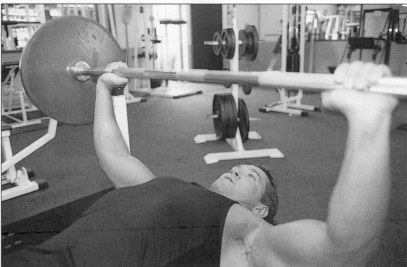

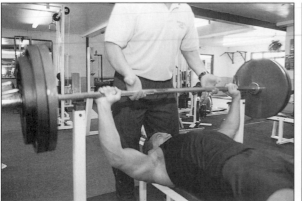

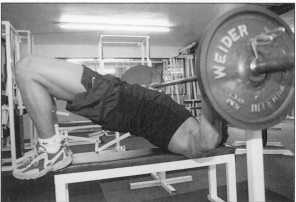

Figure 1

Figure 2

## INCLINE BENCH PRESS

Lie on an incline bench with the backrest at 45 degrees. Keep your back on the bench and your feet on the floor. Grip the bar-bell with your palms facing your feet and your arms shoulder-width apart. Your eyes should be almost directly under the bar. The rack should be at a level that forces you to bend your arms before lifting the bar from it. Take the weight of the bar-bell and lock it out so that your arms are at 90 degrees to the floor. Lower the bar-bell slowly until it lightly touches your chest, ensuring that you keep your elbows pointed outwards. Hold it for a second after the downward phase, before slowly raising the bar-bell over your chest again.

**FORM GUIDE:** Change the degree of incline to hit different areas of your upper pectorals. Try not to arch your back. If you find that you can't help but do this, you need to take the weight down. Keep your hips and head solidly on the bench, and don't attempt to bounce the bar-bell off your chest.

**MUSCLES TARGETED:** Pectorals, tricep, deltoid.

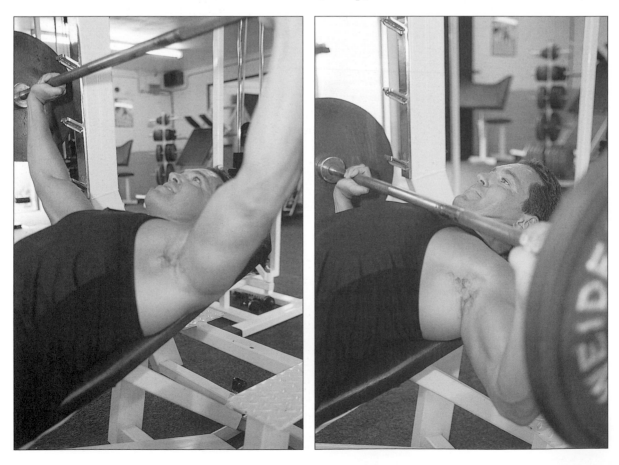

# DUMB-BELL PULLOVERS

Lie at a right angle on a weight bench so that only your shoulders are in contact with the bench. Your feet should be flat on the floor. Holding a dumb-bell with both hands above your chest, keep your arms extended and lower the weight down in an arc behind your head. At this point you should feel your chest and ribcage stretch. When the dumb-bell is as low as you can get it, bring it back up through the same arc to the starting position.

**FORM GUIDE:** Ensure that you keep your hips pushed down towards the floor – this will increase the stretch and focus on the targeted muscles. This is usually the last chest exercise I do, as I find it helps me stretch out the whole of my chest.

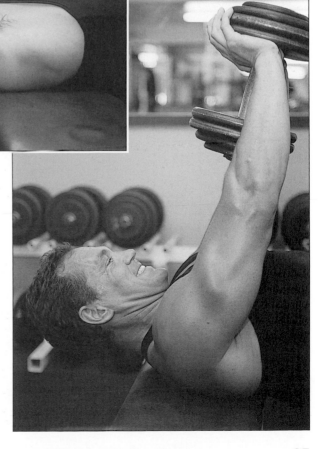

**MUSCLES TARGETED:**
Pectoral.

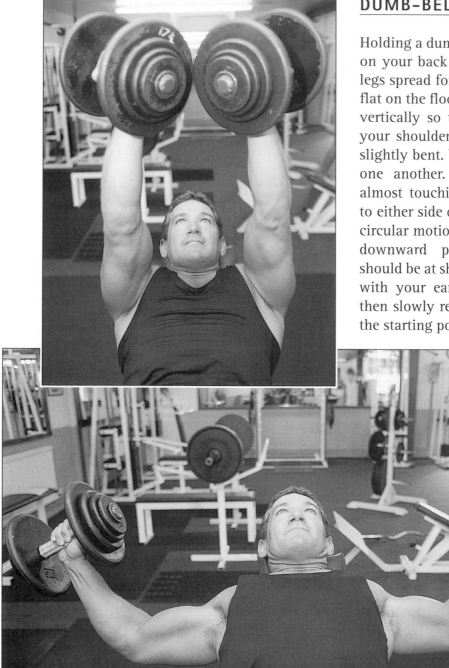

## DUMB-BELL FLYES

Holding a dumb-bell in each hand, lie on your back on the exercise bench, legs spread for stability and your feet flat on the floor. Raise the dumb-bells vertically so that they're just above your shoulders and your elbows are slightly bent. Your palms should face one another. With the dumb-bells almost touching, slowly lower them to either side of your chest in a semi-circular motion. At the bottom of the downward phase the dumb-bells should be at shoulder level and in line with your ears. Hold for a second, then slowly return the dumb-bells to the starting position.

**FORM GUIDE:** Heavy weights make it very difficult to maintain good from initially so start with light weights and build. Use the narrowest bench you can find so that you can pinch your shoulder blades together more easily and your arms are free to move on the downward phase of the exercise. This means that your pectorals are stretched better, making the contraction phase more effective.

As a change, try the exercise on an incline bench to hit your upper pectorals harder. Just make sure that you keep your feet planted firmly on the floor, otherwise you'll upset your balance and fall off the bench (see Figure 1).

**MUSCLES TARGETED:** Pectoral, deltoid.

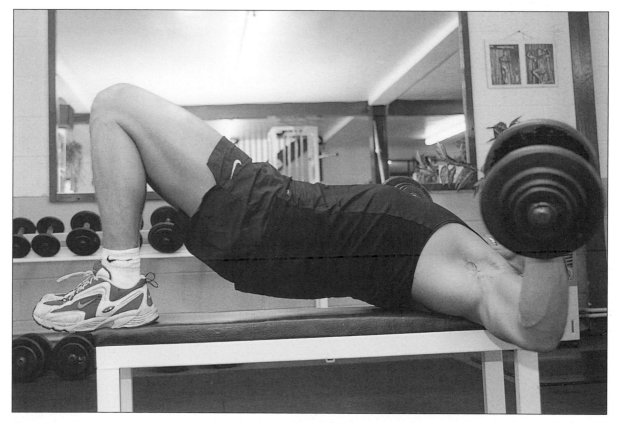

*Figure 1*

## DIPS

Facing a set of dip bars, grab the handles and press your body up so that your arms are fully extended, and cross your legs behind you at the ankle. Keep your knees bent and try not to lock out your elbows. Slowly lower your body by bending your arms. Go as far down as you comfortably can or until your elbows form a right angle, hold the position for a moment, then press yourself back up.

**FORM GUIDE:** Try not to swing your body during the movement. When you are on the upward movement make sure that your elbows don't lock out fully before you lower yourself again.

**MUSCLES TARGETED:** Pectoral, tricep, rhomboid.

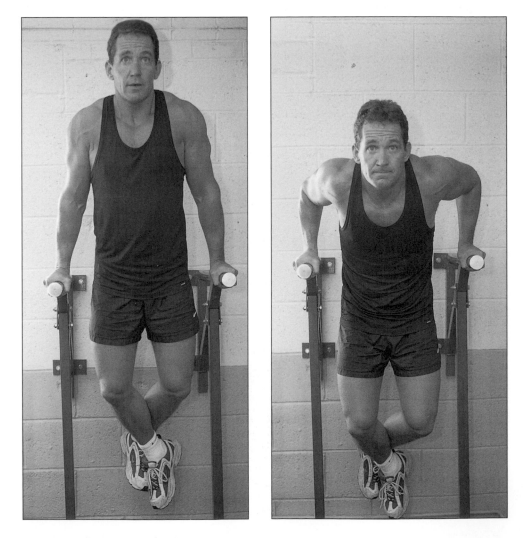

# ii) Legs

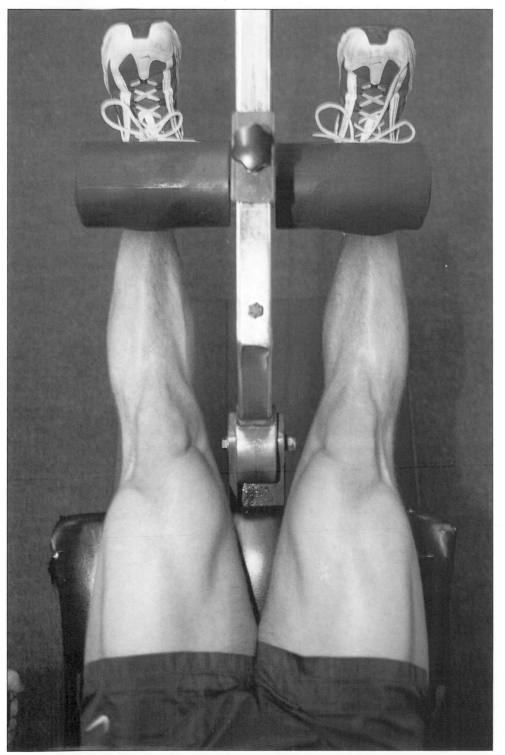

## SQUATS

This exercise hits a stack of muscles in one go, but is predominantly a lower-body exercise. Use a spotter or bar-bell rack to help you get a bar-bell across your upper back and shoulders, and grip it with your hands slightly more than shoulder-width apart, palms facing away from your body. Stand up straight and distribute the weight evenly on to both feet. Tense your back muscles and relax your knees, then sink slowly into a knee-bend. Don't drop your head; it should be in line with your torso with your eyes looking ahead. Concentrate on lowering your hips so that your knees come forward as you squat down. Don't allow your knees to extend past the line of your toes, and don't let your rear go lower than your knees. Continue the movement until your thighs are parallel to the floor. Slowly rise to the starting position.

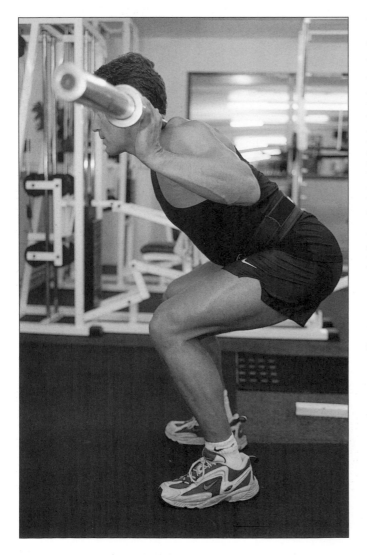

**FORM GUIDE:** When you are starting out, practise the exercise using an un-weighted bar until you are familiar with the form. Make sure you're not leaning too far forward as this will put too much pressure on your back (see Figure 1). To keep your back in line and your torso straight, look at a point in front of you that is slightly above eye level. As the weight gets heavier it is essential that you do the exercise from a bar-bell rack or use a spotter, so that you can pick up and relieve yourself of the bar easily and safely.

**MUSCLES TARGETED:**
Quadricep, gluteal, hamstring, soleus, erector spinae, abdominal.

*Figure 1*

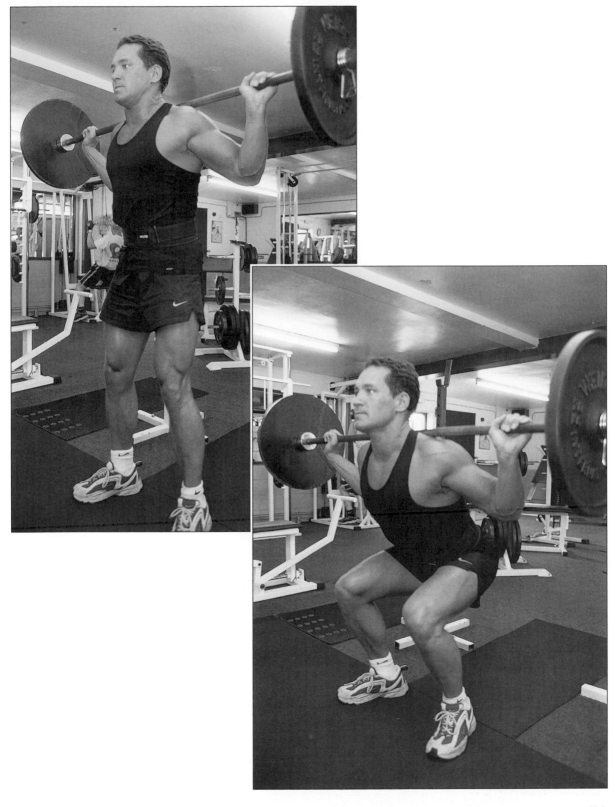

## SMITH–MACHINE SQUATS

In the standing position, place your shoulders under the bar with your feet shoulder-width apart. Squat down, bending your knees until your thighs are parallel to the floor, then press back up to the starting position.

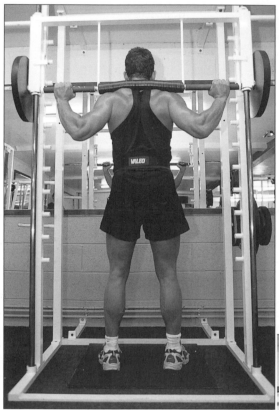

**FORM GUIDE:** I prefer to do squats on a Smith machine because you can work your thighs intensely while putting less strain on other areas such as your lower back and knees. By turning your toes out slightly, you will target the inside of your thigh, and by pointing them in, you will target your outer thighs. If you place your feet slightly in front of your shoulders you will isolate the quadriceps, concentrating on the area nearest the knee – this will also cut down on any excess strain on the back.

**MUSCLES TARGETED:** Quadricep, gluteal, hamstring, soleus, erector spinae, abdominal.

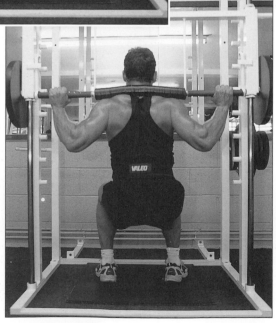

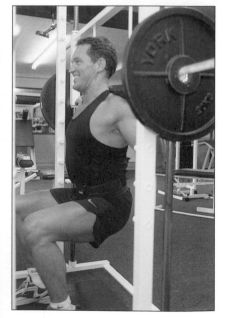

# LEG PRESS MACHINE

Sit in a leg press machine, making sure the seat height is adjusted so that your knees are bent at 90 degrees. On the foot plate, your feet should be as far apart as your hips. Push forward on the foot plate to straighten your legs, keeping your knees unlocked. Now slowly return to the starting position.

**FORM GUIDE:** Putting your feet in different areas on the foot plate will work different muscles. With your feet together, you'll be exercising your hamstring; placing them around two feet apart will work the inside of the hamstrings, groin and gluteal muscles. Keep your feet in this position and point your toes out at 45 degrees and you'll create more pressure on the upper areas of the groin and backside. Placing them shoulder-width apart will exercise the front of the quadriceps.

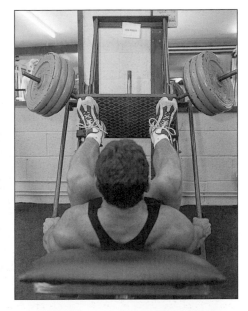

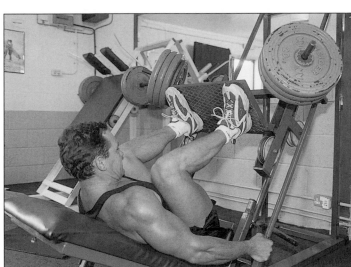

**MUSCLES TARGETED:**
Hamstring, quadricep, gluteal.

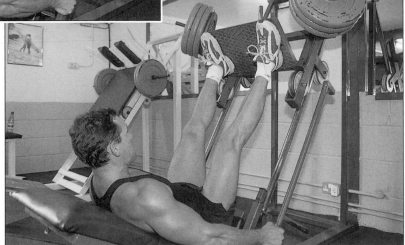

## LYING LEG CURL (HAMSTRINGS)

Lie on your stomach on the machine. With your ankles behind the pads, your knee joints should be in line with the axis of the machine. Your legs should be fully extended, knees slightly bent. Grip the handles or the side of the bench. Now lift the leg pad as high as possible in a controlled motion, keeping your pelvis pushed into the bench. When your heels are at an angle just under 90 degrees, slowly return to the starting position.

**FORM GUIDE:** If you find there's a bit too much pressure on your lower back, roll up a towel and place it under your hips as you lie down on the machine. Use your toes to concentrate the pressure on different muscles in the hamstring and calf. Turning your toes out will work more of the calf muscles and outer thigh area of the hamstrings. Turning your toes in, with your feet flexed, works more of the inner thighs in the hamstring area.

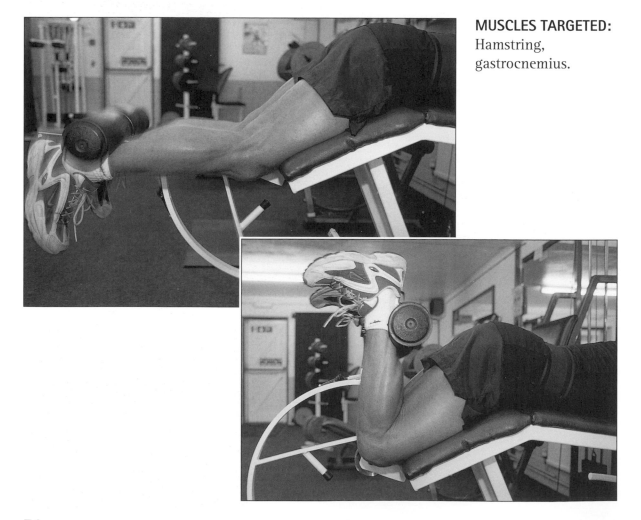

**MUSCLES TARGETED:** Hamstring, gastrocnemius.

## LEG EXTENSION

I use these as a warm-up for my legs before I go into my squats. Sit in a leg extension machine with your legs behind the pads. Your knees should be at the axis of the machine. Make sure your back is fully supported against the pad, your hands gripping the handles. Bend your feet towards your shins to consolidate your knee joints throughout the exercise and bend your knees at slightly more than a 90-degree angle. Raise your legs with a controlled motion until they are almost straight, keeping your knees unlocked. Hold for a second at the top of the movement. Slowly return to the starting position.

**FORM GUIDE:** Make sure that the targeted muscles are under constant tension by maintaining a constant speed throughout. For maximum pressure, hold for four seconds at the top of each extension. Turning your toes out will work more of the inner quadricep muscles and vice versa.

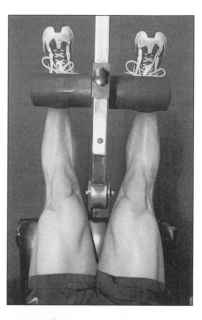

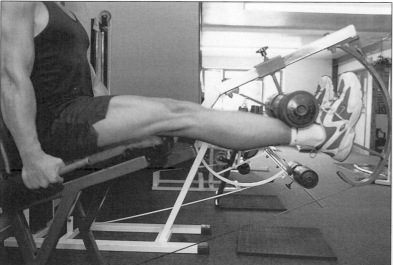

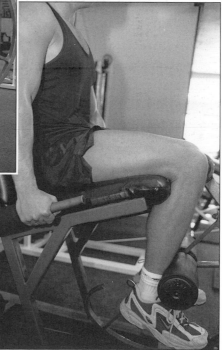

**MUSCLES TARGETED:** Quadricep.

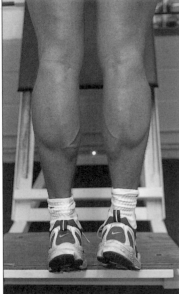

## MACHINE CALF RAISES (STANDING AND SEATED)

Stand on the step of the calf machine with your hands on the grips. Keep your legs slightly bent to begin with, and place your toes and the balls of your feet a few inches apart on the edge of the step. Raise your heels with a controlled motion as far as they will go so that the machine's weight is transmitted to your shoulders via the pads. Keep your legs bent and try not to lock out your knees. Lower your body slowly back to the starting position until you feel the weight of the machine release from your shoulders.

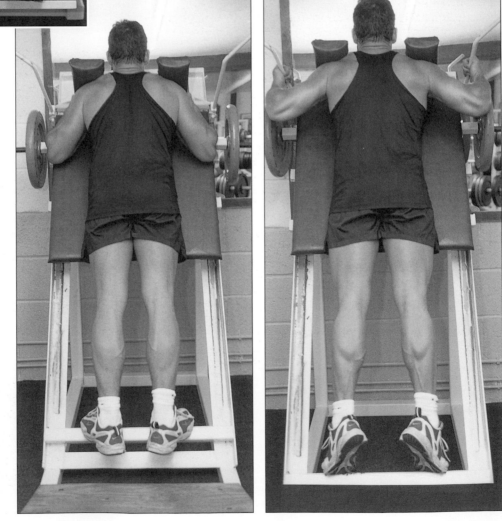

**FORM GUIDE:** Don't vary the position of the balls of your feet during the exercise, keeping strain off the knee joints and on the targeted muscles. For variation try seated calf raises where you sit on the machine and place the balls of your feet on the bottom step with your knees planted firmly under the padded T-bar. Slowly lower your heels as far down as possible, and then press back up on your toes until your calves are fully contracted.

**MUSCLES TARGETED:** Gastrocnemius, soleus.

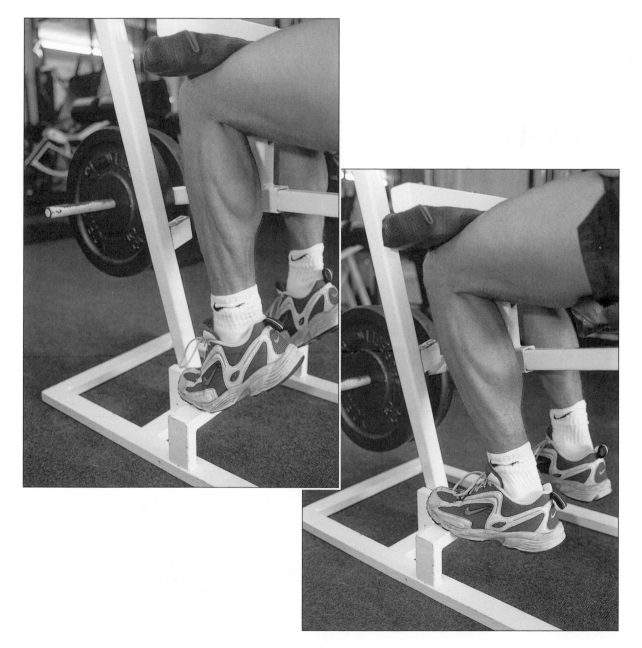

# iii) Back

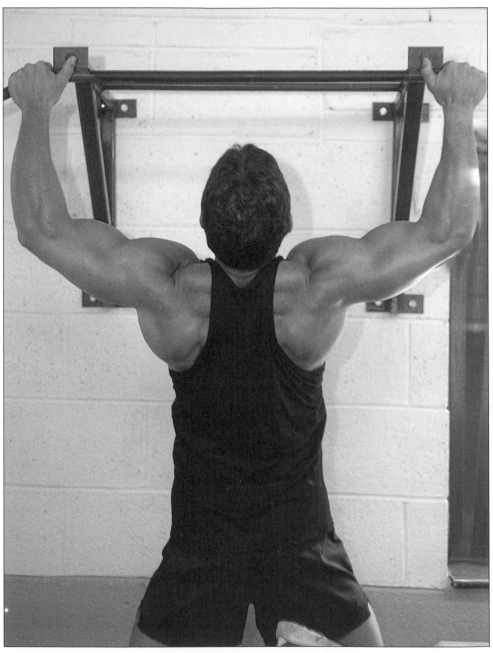

## SEATED CABLE ROWS

Keep your back straight as you lean forward and break at the waist, grabbing the handles and pulling the cable back. Your body should be leaning forward with your arms fully extended. Bring the handles in until they touch your chest and your upper body is now in an upright position. Your elbows should be pointing behind you and your knees should be unlocked. Hold for a second and then return to the starting position.

**FORM GUIDE:** Reduce risk of injury by keeping your back straight at all times. The wider your grip, the more your mid and lower back are worked; the narrower the grip, the more the upper back is worked.

**MUSCLES TARGETED:**
Latissimus dorsi, trapezius, rhomboid, deltoid, bicep.

## BENT-OVER BAR-BELL ROWS

This is another compound exercise which will hit a lot of muscles in one go. Stand with your feet hip-width apart, knees slightly bent. Bend forward until your upper body is parallel with the floor. At this point it's essential to keep your back straight. Let the bar hang at arm's length in front of you, just in front of your legs. Lift the bar upwards until it touches the upper part of your stomach, then lower it again with a controlled motion until you're back at the starting position.

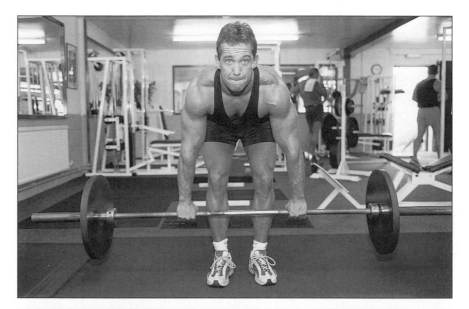

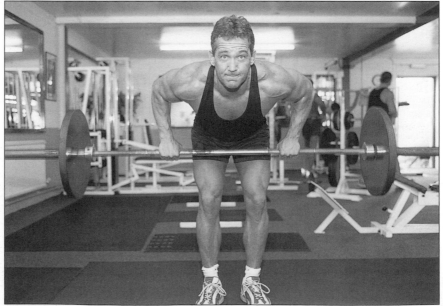

**FORM GUIDE:** Throughout the exercise the body must not move. Make sure the bar-bell is lowered with a controlled motion, and is not allowed to drop forward.

**MUSCLES TARGETED:** Latissimus dorsi, trapezius, rhomboid, deltoid.

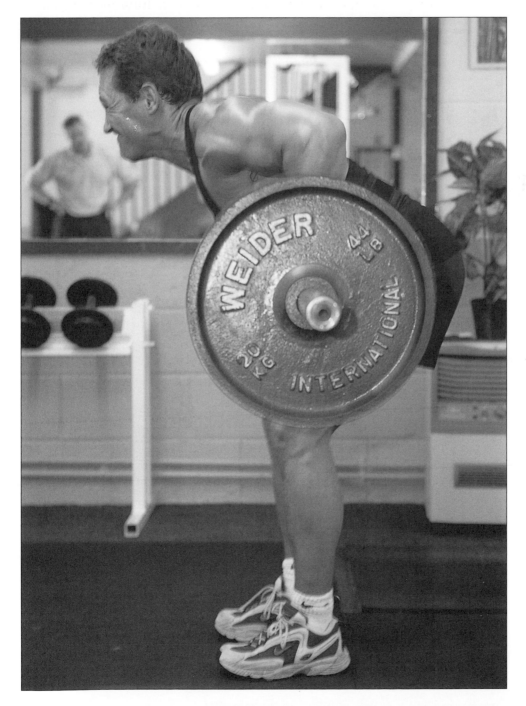

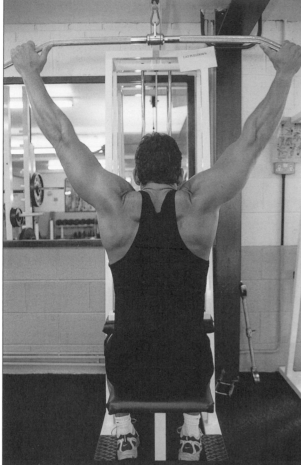

## LATERAL PULL-DOWN

Adjust the knee pad on the machine so that your knees fit under it while bent at 90 degrees. Make sure that you can lift your heels by about an inch. Wrap your hands around the bar with a grip that's about six inches wider than your shoulders on each side. This usually means gripping the bar just at the point where it becomes angled, just past the bend. Bring the bar down behind your head, until it almost touches the top of your back. Make sure that as you let the bar back up you stop the motion before your arms fully extend.

**FORM GUIDE:** As a variant, you can pull the bar to the front of your chest or you can attach different bars to give you different grips (see Figures 1 & 2). Keep your upper body stationary. Make sure that your feet stay on the floor throughout, as thrashing

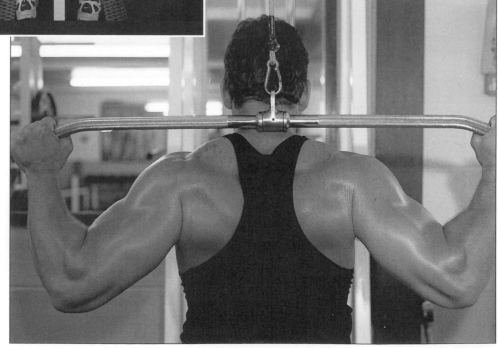

them about in a fight for more leverage will only ruin your form, decrease the benefits of the exercise and increase the risk of a back injury.

**MUSCLES TARGETED:** Trapezius, rhomboid.

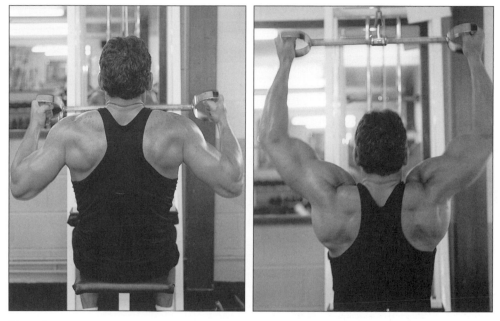

*Figure 1*

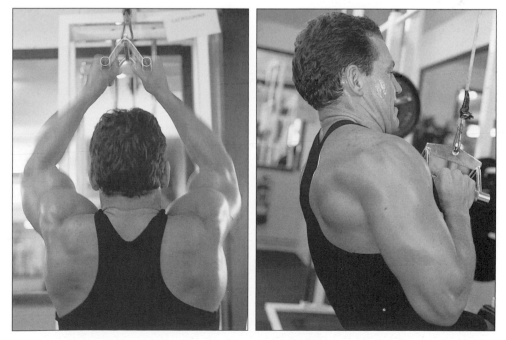

*Figure 2*

## ONE-ARM DUMB-BELL ROWS

Put your left leg on one end of an exercise bench and your left hand on the other end. Your upper body should be roughly parallel with the ground. Plant your right leg firmly on the floor to the side of the bench. Hold a dumb-bell with your right hand, palm facing inwards. Bend your arm slightly and lift the dumb-bell to your torso. Your elbow will move backwards and upwards, and you'll need to raise your shoulder as high as possible. Your forearm should remain pointing at the floor at all times. Hold for a second, then lower the dumb-bell to the starting position. After you've finished your set, swap sides.

**FORM GUIDE:** Keep your arm close to your body throughout the exercise and concentrate on the correct positioning of your elbow to maintain good form.

**MUSCLES TARGETED:**
Latissimus dorsi, trapezius, rhomboid, deltoid.

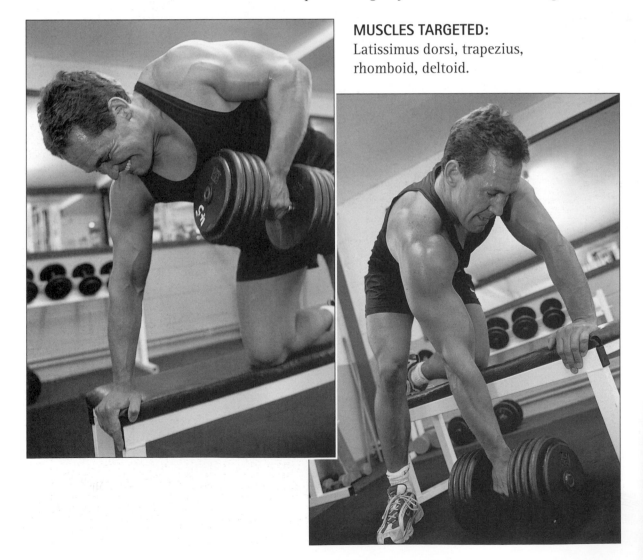

# DUMB-BELL SHRUGS

Stand with your feet shoulder-width apart, with two heavy dumb-bells in each hand. Raise your shoulders as high up as possible and try to touch your ears. Hold in this position for a moment, then return to the starting position.

**FORM GUIDE:** Try not to move anything but your shoulders. As a variant, you can also perform the exercise with a bar-bell.

**MUSCLES TARGETED:** Trapezius.

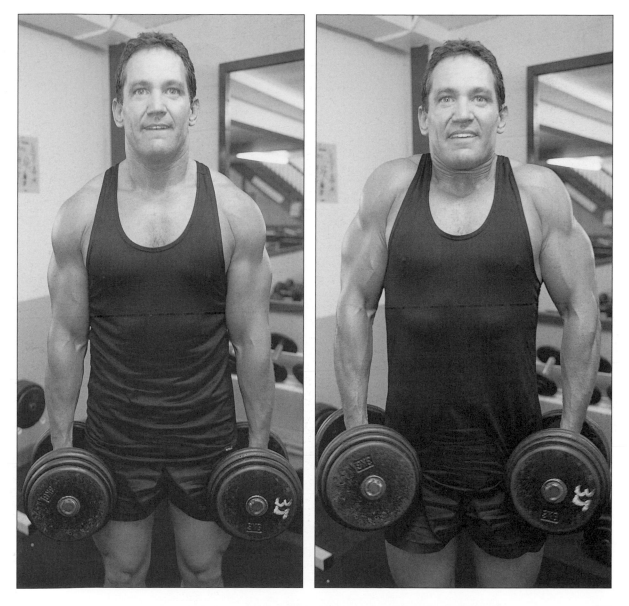

## CHIN-UPS

I usually start my back routine with these because it opens my back muscles up and stretches them thoroughly. Perform your set with your hands shoulder-width apart, and with an overhand grip (your palms facing away from you). Hang from the bar with your ankles crossed. Slowly pull yourself up until your chin is over the bar. Hold for a second, then lower yourself to the starting position.

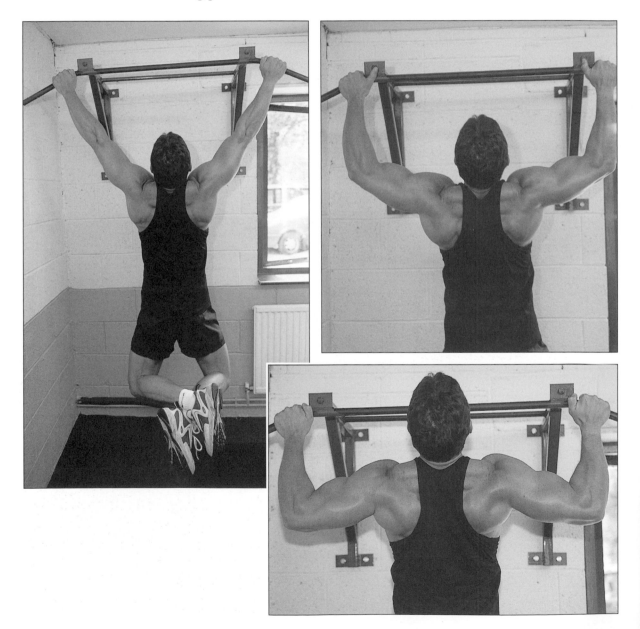

**FORM GUIDE:** As a variant, change to an underhand grip with your hands about two inches apart. This will target the lower part of your back and place more emphasis on your biceps (see Figures 1, 2 & 3). Don't stop at the bottom of the movement, go immediately into your next pull-up.

**MUSCLES TARGETED:** Rhomboid, trapezius, supraspinatus, pectoral, bicep.

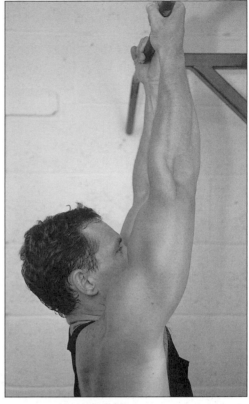

*Figure 2*

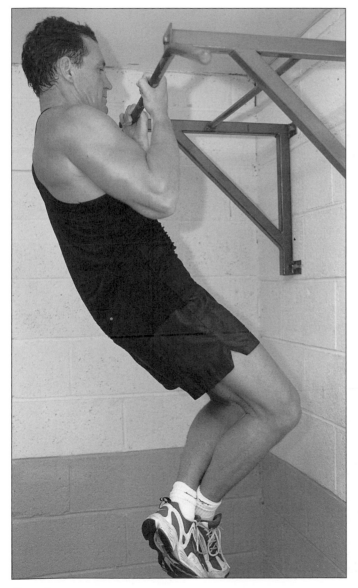

*Figure 1*

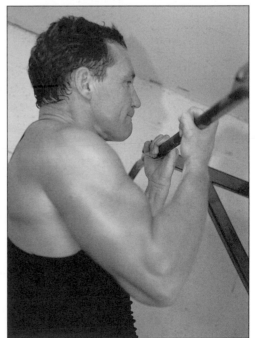

*Figure 3*

# iv) Shoulders

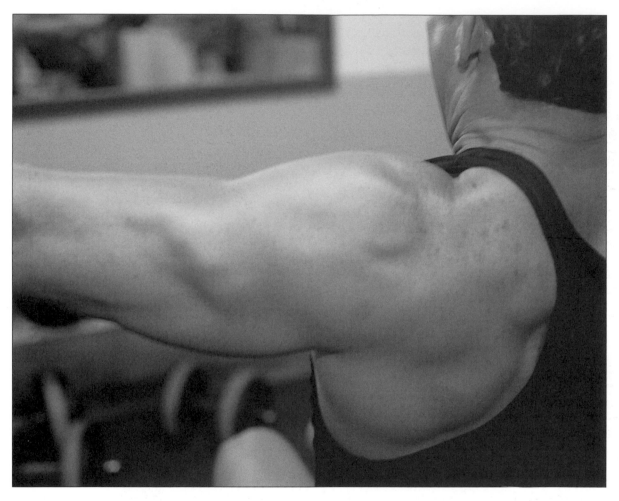

## MILITARY PRESS

Stand with your back straight, feet shoulder-width apart and knees slightly bent. Using an overhand grip, hold a bar-bell with your hands shoulder-width apart or slightly wider. Bend your elbows and bring the bar up to shoulder level so that your palms end up facing the ceiling while your elbows point down. This is the starting position. Slowly lift the bar straight over your head. Hold for a second, then slowly lower to the chest again.

**FORM GUIDE:** Start with a light weight until you get familiar with the form and don't bounce the bar off your chest. If you find that you're swaying when you raise the bar, use a lighter weight until you can lift with complete control.

If you have back problems you can do a seated version of the same exercise on a weight bench. The form is exactly the same, but remember to keep your back and head pressed against the backrest.

**MUSCLES TARGETED:** Deltoid, trapezius, supraspinatus, pectoral, tricep.

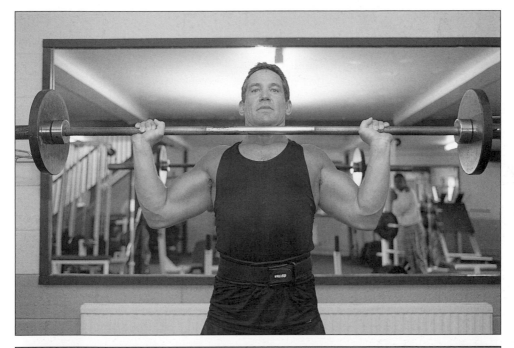

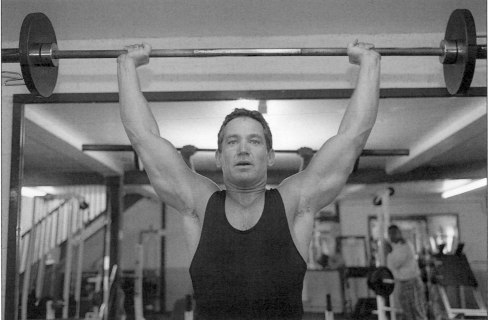

## SEATED DUMB-BELL PRESS

Sit on a weight bench with your back supported, a dumb-bell in each hand with your palms facing your body at shoulder height. Slowly raise the dumb-bells until they almost touch above your head. Straighten your arms but don't lock out your elbows completely. Hold for a second, then lower the dumb-bells to the starting position.

**FORM GUIDE:** To maintain the pressure on your targeted muscles, keep your body as still as possible throughout the exercise. If you find yourself swaying or jerking the weight up into the air, you should think about bringing the weight down a little.

**MUSCLES TARGETED:** Deltoid, tricep, trapezius.

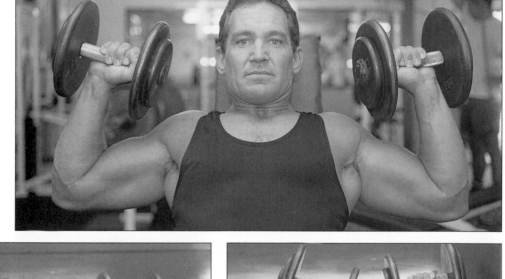

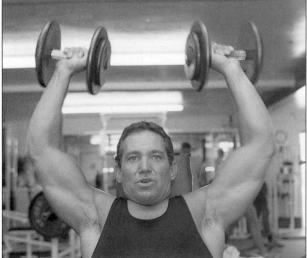

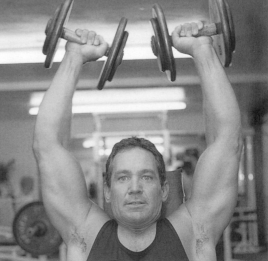

## STANDING LATERAL RAISE

Hold a dumb-bell in each hand, with your arms down by your sides and your palms facing your body. Stand straight, with your feet shoulder-width apart and your knees slightly bent. Lean forward slightly at the waist, keeping your shoulders, neck and back straight. Lift your arms evenly in a semicircle to your shoulders. Don't raise the weights above your shoulders. Your palms should now be facing the floor. Throughout the movement your arms should be slightly bent (if you lock your elbows you'll put too much strain on your elbow joints), but you should try and keep your arms in line with your body and your wrists in line with your forearms. Hold for a second, then slowly lower your arms to the starting position.

**FORM GUIDE:** Keep the movements smooth and controlled; jerking your arms up in an effort for greater momentum will only reduce the effectiveness of the exercise. Keep your head in line with your spine at all times. To target the muscles, concentrate on squeezing your deltoids as you raise your arms.

**MUSCLES TARGETED:** Deltoid.

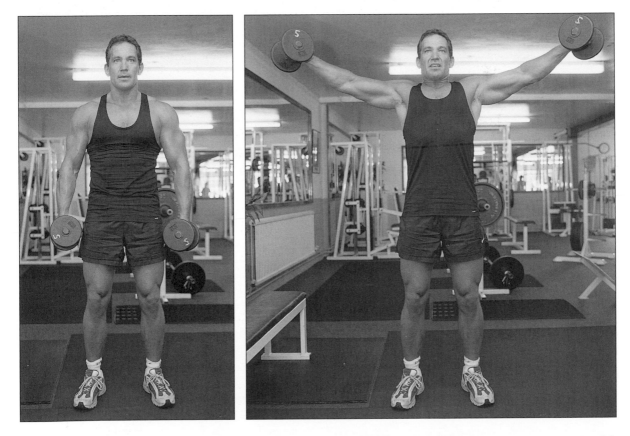

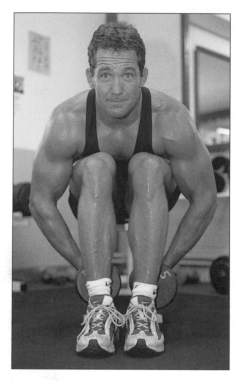

## SEATED BENT-OVER LATERAL RAISE

Sit down on a weight bench, holding a dumb-bell in each hand, with your arms hanging naturally in front of you. Your hands will be under your legs, with your palms facing one another. Raise both arms at the same time in a controlled, circular movement until they reach shoulder level. Hold for a second, then lower to the starting position.

**FORM GUIDE:** Your arms should stay slightly bent throughout the exercise, and keep your chest as close to your thighs as is comfortable.

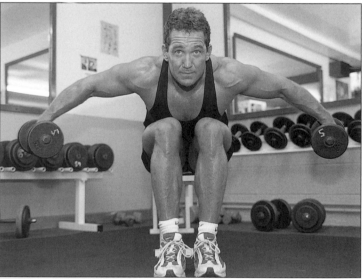

**MUSCLES TARGETED:**
Deltoid, trapezius, rhomboid.

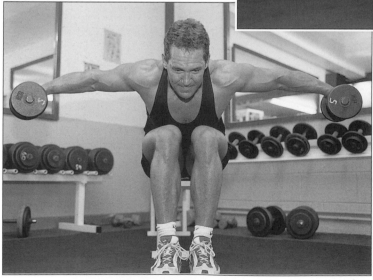

## UPRIGHT ROW

Stand with your feet parallel and shoulder-width apart. Hold a bar-bell or EZ curl bar, with your palms facing your legs and your arms shoulder-width apart. The bar should be resting on your upper thighs. Lean forward slightly at the waist and allow your shoulders to drop forward, but keep your back straight. Now pull the bar-bell upwards towards your collarbone, following the vertical line of your body but not touching it. Your elbows should be

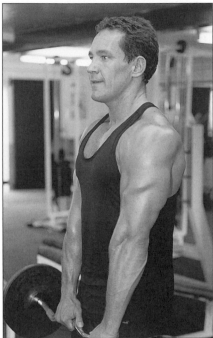

pointing outwards and above the bar-bell. Hold for a second, then return the bar to the starting position.

**FORM GUIDE:** It's important not to lean back or sway when lifting the bar as this makes the exercise easier and dramatically reduces the effect it has on the targeted muscles. On the upward phase imagine your elbows being pulled upwards and outwards. On the downward phase your elbows should be the last thing to be lowered.

**MUSCLES TARGETED:** Deltoid, trapezius, rhomboid, bicep.

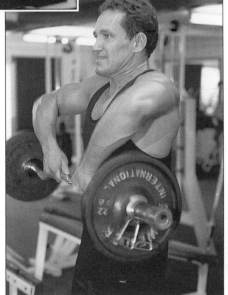

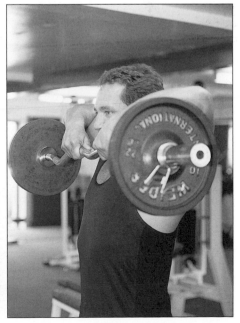

# v) Arms (biceps)

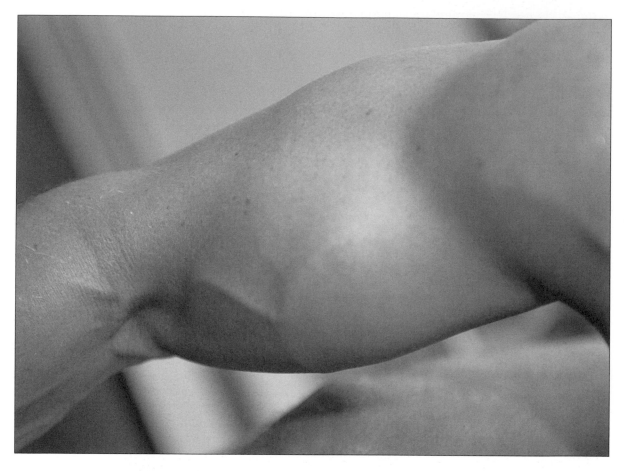

## STANDING BAR-BELL CURL

This exercise is a great springboard to strength and confidence if you're new to weights or are coming back after a long lay-off. Stand with your feet shoulder-width apart and your knees slightly bent. With your arms fully extended, grip the bar-bell with your palms facing upwards and spaced slightly wider than your shoulders. Curl the bar-bell up towards your neck, hold for a second at the top of this phase, then lower the bar to the starting position.

**FORM GUIDE:** For a variant, grip the bar with your hands two to three inches apart in a narrow-grip – it's a good idea to use an EZ curl bar to take the strain off your wrist (see Figures 1 & 2, page 96). Keep the bar-bell under control using only your biceps, and don't swing it erratically during the

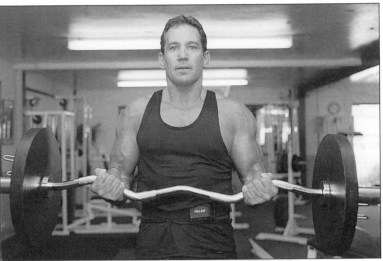

movement (see Figures 3 & 4, page 96). Protect your elbow joints by resisting the temptation to jerk the bar-bell back up at the bottom of the curl, which would also lessen the results of the exercise on the targeted muscles. If you're having difficulty doing this, stand with your back against a wall and keep your upper body straight.

**MUSCLES TARGETED:** Bicep.

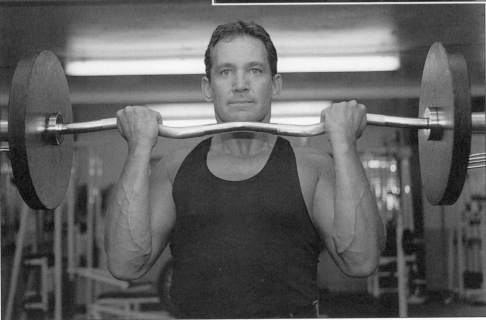

*Continued*

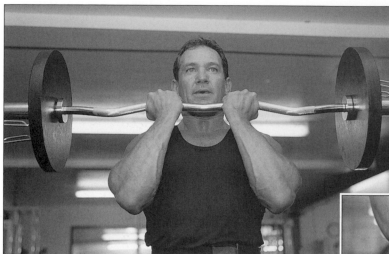

*Figure 1*

*Figure 2*

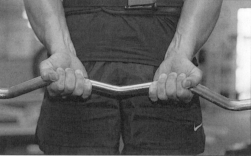

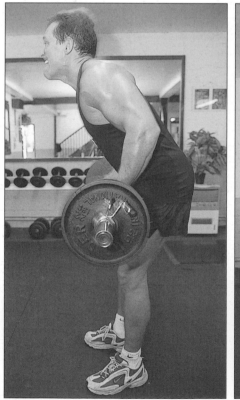

*Figure 3*

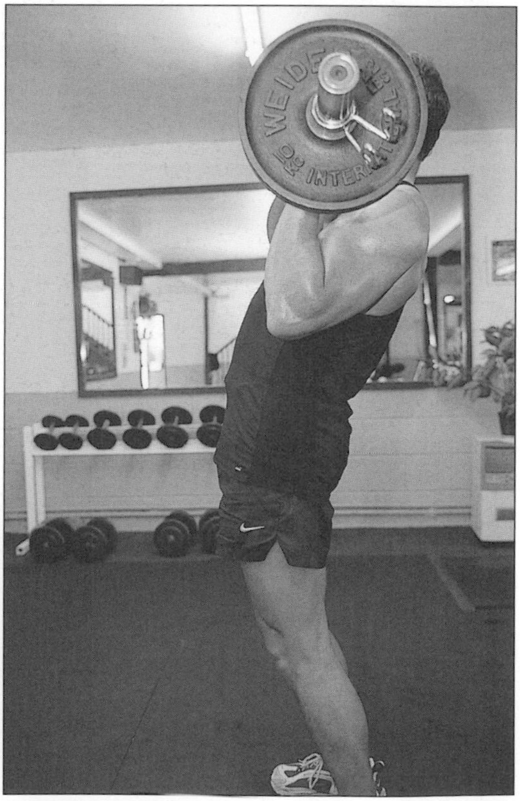

*Figure 4*

THE EXERCISES • STANDING BAR-BELL CURL

# INCLINE SEATED DUMB-BELL CURL

Sit back on an incline bench holding a dumb-bell in each hand, with your arms at your sides, palms facing inwards. Slowly curl the right dumb-bell up towards your neck turning your arm as you do so – the back of your hand should end up facing outwards. This twisting motion ensures that the exercise works the forearm as well as the bicep. Hold for a second, then lower the dumb-bell to the starting position. Repeat with the opposite arm.

**FORM GUIDE:** Keep your upper arms tight to your body, and your elbows stationary throughout. The more you twist your wrist on the upward phase of the lift, the more it will focus the exercise on the targeted muscles. After a few weeks, aim to finish at the top of the lift with your palms facing as far to the side of your body as is comfortable.

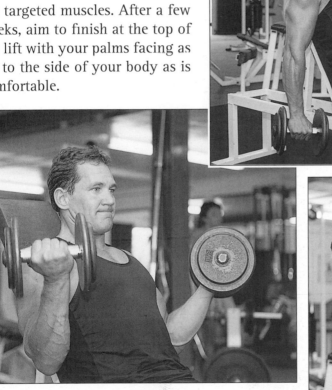

**MUSCLES TARGETED:** Bicep.

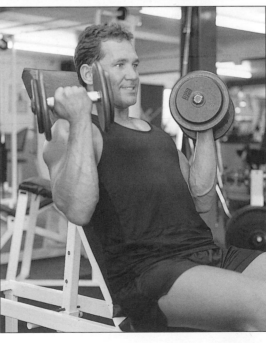

## STANDING DUMB-BELL CURL

Stand with your feet shoulder-width apart, with a dumb-bell in each hand. Slowly curl the right dumb-bell up towards your neck, turning your arm as you do so the back of your hand ends up facing outwards. This twisting motion ensures that the exercise works the forearm as well as the bicep. Hold for a second, then lower the dumb-bell to the starting position. Repeat with the opposite arm.

**FORM GUIDE:** Keep your upper arms tight to your body and your elbows stationary throughout. The more you twist your wrist on the upward phase of the lift, the more it will focus the exercise on the targeted muscles. After a few weeks, aim to finish at the top of the lift with your palms facing as far to the side of your body as is comfortable.

**MUSCLES TARGETED:** Bicep.

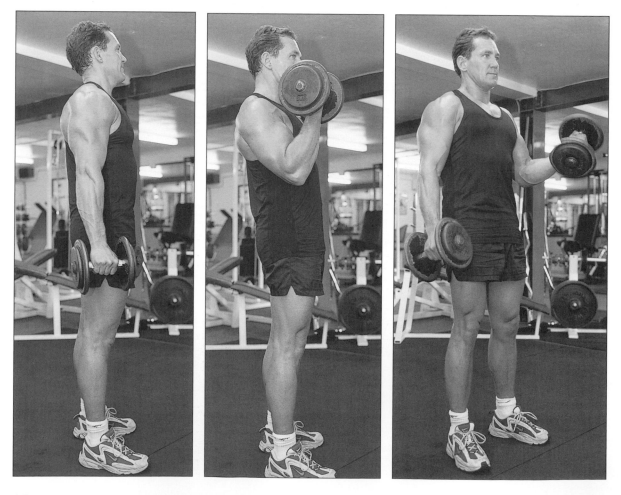

## STANDING CABLE CURL

Stand about a foot away from the machine, and hold the grip with both hands, palms facing upwards. Keep your elbows tucked into your body and slowly curl the pulley grip upwards. Hold for a second at the end of this phase, and then return the grip slowly to the starting position.

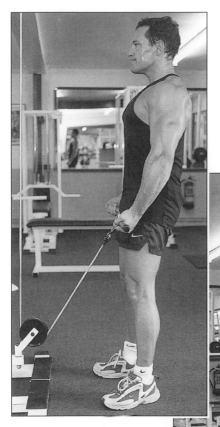

**FORM GUIDE:** Resist the force of the machine, which will pull you towards it, by keeping your chest pushed out and your shoulders back.

**MUSCLES TARGETED:** Bicep, brachialis, brachioradialis.

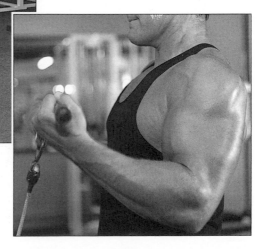

## STANDING REVERSE CABLE CURL

Stand about a foot away from the machine and hold the grip with both hands, palms facing downward. Keep your elbows tucked into your body, and slowly curl the pulley grip upwards. Hold for a second at the end of this phase, and then return the grip slowly to the starting position. Now curl your wrists towards your body until you feel a contraction in your forearms.

**FORM GUIDE:** Resist the force of the machine, which will pull you towards it, by keeping your chest pushed out and your shoulders back.

**MUSCLES TARGETED:** Bicep, brachialis, brachioradialis.

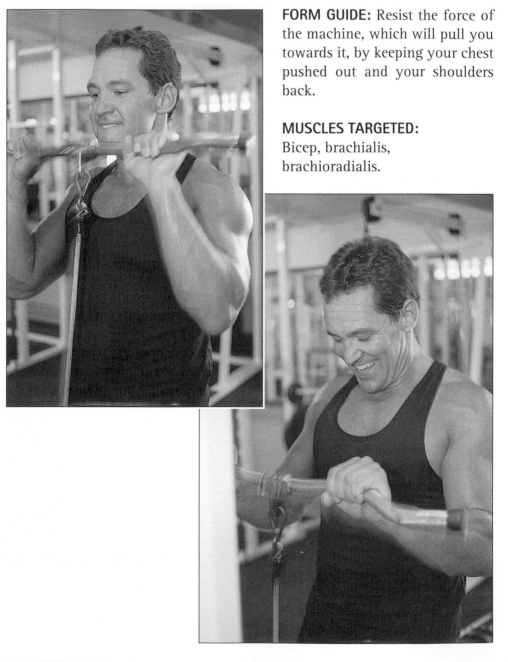

# vi) Arms (triceps)

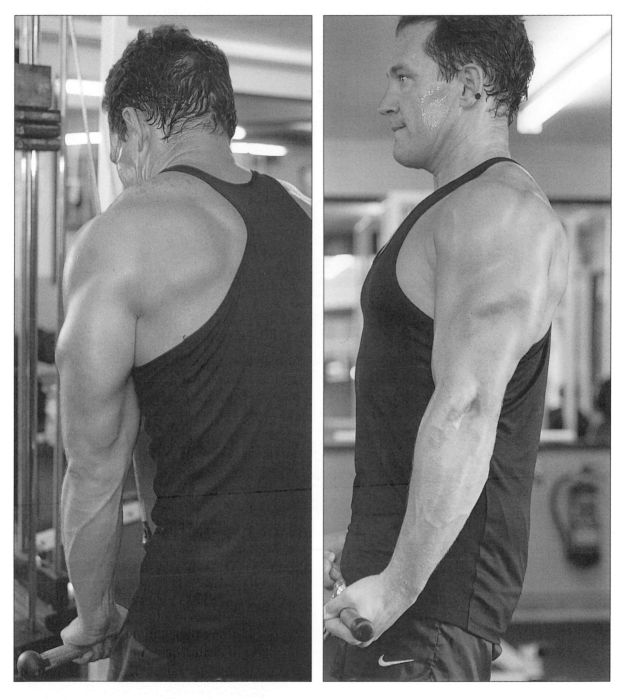

## CABLE PUSH-DOWNS

Adjust the pulley of a cable machine so that it's at the top of its setting. Stand facing the machine, holding the bar at chest height with both hands in a narrow grip, palms facing down. Your legs should be shoulder-width apart and your knees slightly bent. Keeping your elbows and upper arms tucked into your body, extend both your elbows, pressing the bar down as far as you can. Keep your wrists straight and hold the bar for a second at the downward phase of the exercise. Now allow the bar to rise back to the starting position slowly and under full control.

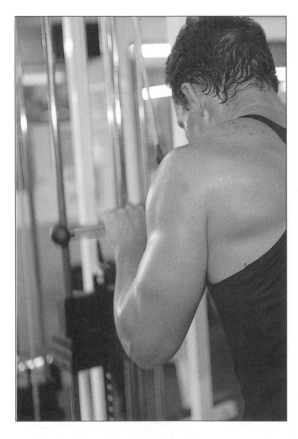

**FORM GUIDE:** Push down only with your arms, don't let your upper body help you with the weight. Change the handles occasionally to work the targeted muscle at a slightly different angle.

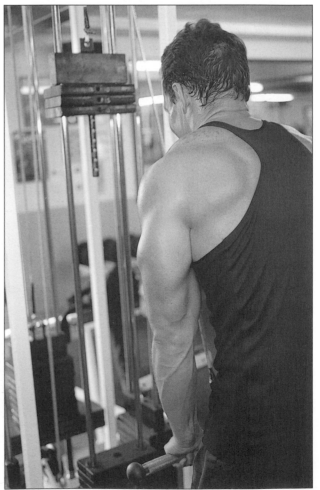

**MUSCLES TARGETED:**
Tricep.

## CABLE ROPE PUSH-DOWNS

Replace the bar with a rope and adjust the pulley of a cable machine so that it's at the top of its setting. Stand facing the machine, holding the rope at chest height with both hands, palms facing and thumbs uppermost in a narrow grip. Your legs should be shoulder-width apart and your knees slightly bent. Keeping your elbows and upper arms tucked into your body, extend both your elbows, pressing the rope down as far as you can. Keep your wrists straight and hold the rope for a second at the downward phase of the exercise. Now allow the rope to rise back to the starting position slowly and under full control.

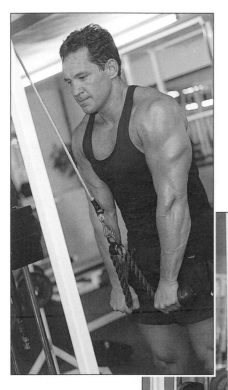

**FORM GUIDE:** Push down only with your arms, don't let your upper body help you with the weight. Keep your back straight throughout the exercise and don't try to gain more leverage by arching your spine and allowing your elbows to come away from your body (see Figure 1).

**MUSCLES TARGETED:** Tricep.

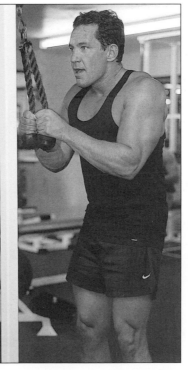

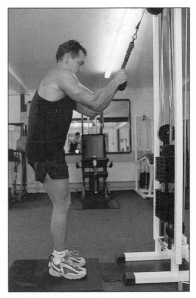

*Figure 1*

## REVERSE-GRIP CABLE PUSH-DOWNS

Adjust the pulley of a cable machine so that it's at the top of its setting. Stand facing the machine, holding the bar at chest height with both hands in a narrow grip, palms facing upwards. Your legs should be shoulder-width apart and your knees slightly bent. Keeping your elbows and upper arms tucked into your body, extend both your elbows, pressing the bar down as far as you can. Keep your wrists straight and hold the bar for a second at the downward phase of the exercise. Now allow the bar to rise back to the starting position slowly and under full control.

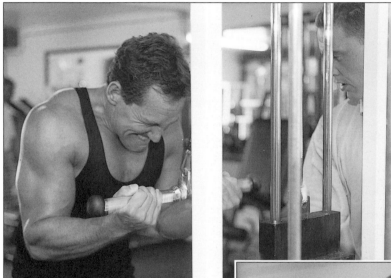

**FORM GUIDE:** Push down only with your arms, don't let your upper body help you with the weight.

**MUSCLES TARGETED:** Tricep.

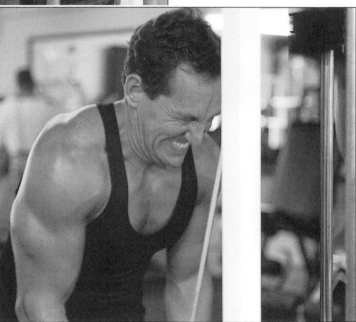

## TRICEP KICKBACK

Holding a dumb-bell in your right hand, rest your left knee and lower leg on a weight bench low enough to keep your back horizontal during the exercise. Stabilise your body by putting your left hand on the edge of the bench. Your upper body should be parallel to the floor, or angled slightly upwards. Bend your right leg and the arm holding the dumb-bell, so that your elbow points to the ceiling and the weight is close to your hip. Now straighten your right arm behind your body, keeping your upper arm parallel to the floor. Hold for a second, then lower to the starting position. Finish your set, then repeat on the left side.

**FORM GUIDE:** It's very difficult to maintain good form and control on this one because you can't call on other muscles to help you perform the lift. But if you keep strict form you'll certainly know that your triceps are doing all the work and getting maximum benefits.

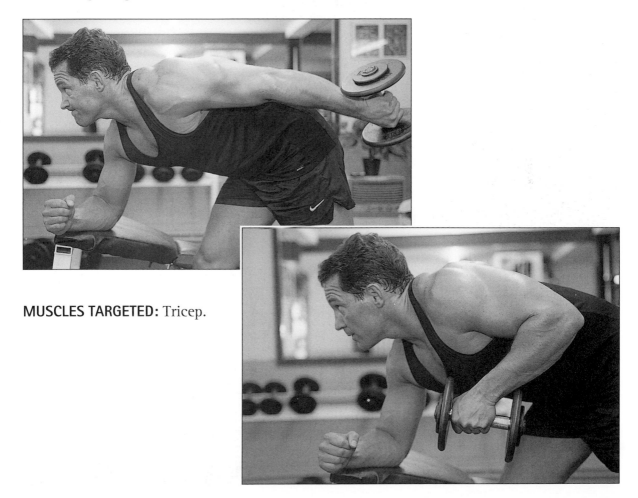

**MUSCLES TARGETED:** Tricep.

## CLOSE-GRIP BENCH PRESS

Lie on the weight bench with your head under the bar-bell rack and your feet flat on the floor. Your hands should be around 12 to 18 inches apart and should let your forearm form a right angle with your upper arm at the bottom of the movement (practise with an imaginary bar-bell). Your wrists should be firm, with your palms facing your feet as you grip the bar. Now lift the bar-bell off the rack and lock it above your chest at arm's length. Slowly bend your elbows, lowering the weight to the middle of your chest. It should touch it gently, more or less in the centre of your breastbone, and your elbows should be below your torso. Hold for a second, then slowly press the bar-bell back up to the starting position.

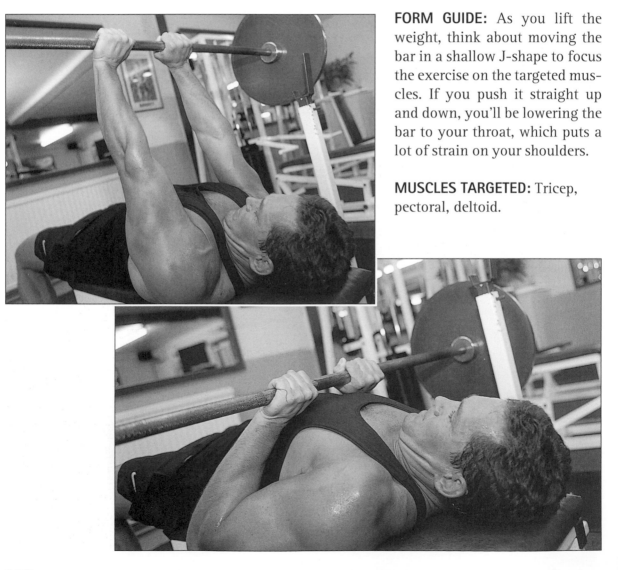

**FORM GUIDE:** As you lift the weight, think about moving the bar in a shallow J-shape to focus the exercise on the targeted muscles. If you push it straight up and down, you'll be lowering the bar to your throat, which puts a lot of strain on your shoulders.

**MUSCLES TARGETED:** Tricep, pectoral, deltoid.

## LYING TRICEP EXTENSION

Lie on a weight bench, knees bent and feet resting on the bench. Hold an EZ curl bar over your chest, with your palms facing away from your face and your arms fully extended. Your hands should be about four to six inches away from one another. Keep your upper arms static but bend your elbows, lowering the bar towards your forehead. Then slowly return the bar to the starting position.

**FORM GUIDE:** This is a difficult exercise, so start with a weight that you know you can manage. Focus on the targeted muscles by making sure not to arch your back or clench your abdominal muscles as you bring the weight back up.

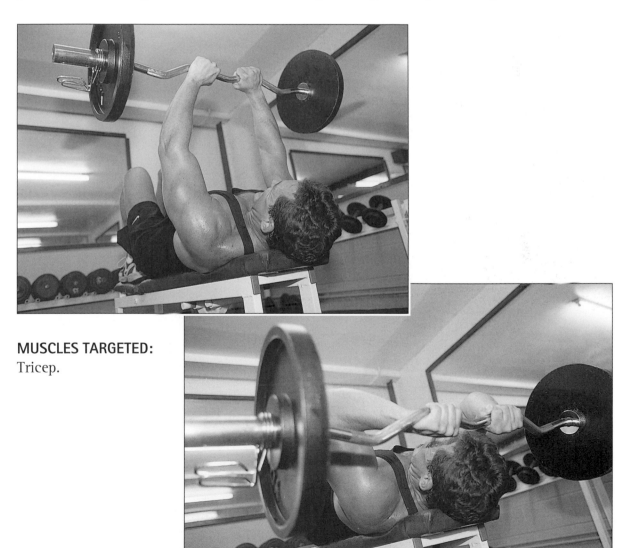

**MUSCLES TARGETED:**
Tricep.

## PRESS-UPS

If you thought you'd left these behind, think again. The press-up is one of the most complete upper-body exercises you can do. You won't need much instruction on this one, but here are a few reminders on technique: your palms should be a little wider than your shoulders; remember that your toes are the pivotal point for the exercise, and your legs and upper body should remain taut and rigid throughout the upward and downward phase of movement.

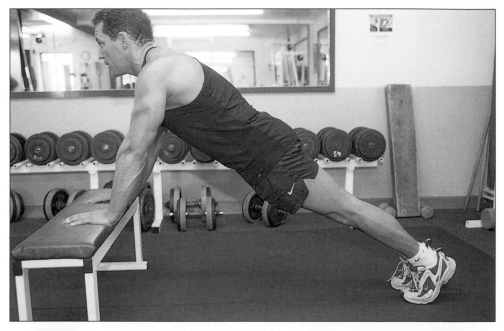

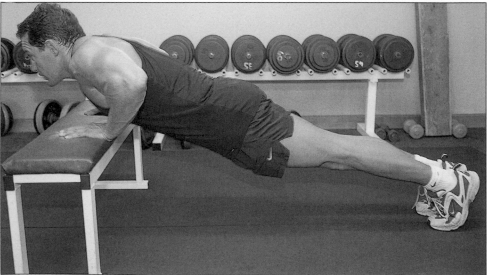

**FORM GUIDE:** For variation, you can place your hands closer together or wider apart. You can also use a weight bench to perform your press-ups at an incline, with your feet or hands resting on the bench. To focus on your chest muscles, move your palms in a few inches.

**MUSCLES TARGETED:** Pectoral, deltoid, bicep, brachialis, brachioradialis, coracobrachialis, tricep.

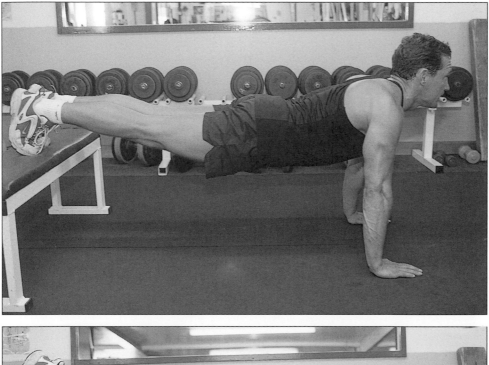

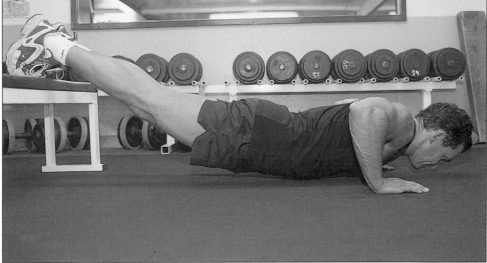

# vii) Abdominals

## INCLINE BOARD CRUNCHES

Lie on your back on an incline bench with your knees bent to take the strain off your lower back and your feet hooked under the supports. Place your hands on your hips or behind your head, but make sure that you don't pull on your head as you raise yourself up. Bring your upper body to 45 degrees, and hold for a second before lowering to the starting position and repeat.

FORM GUIDE: Don't let your back touch the board as you lower yourself back down.

MUSCLES TARGETED: Upper abdominal.

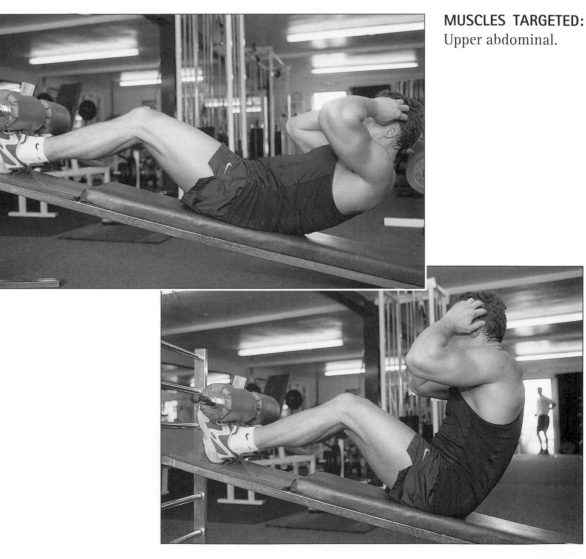

## HANGING LEG RAISES

Hold on to a chinning bar and hang at arm's length. Keeping your legs as straight as you can, lift them up as far as possible, hold for a second, then lower them back to the starting position.

**FORM GUIDE:** Don't swing your feet or allow them to touch the floor during the exercise. If you find this one difficult, try doing it by just lifting your knees up.

**MUSCLES TARGETED:** All the abdominals.

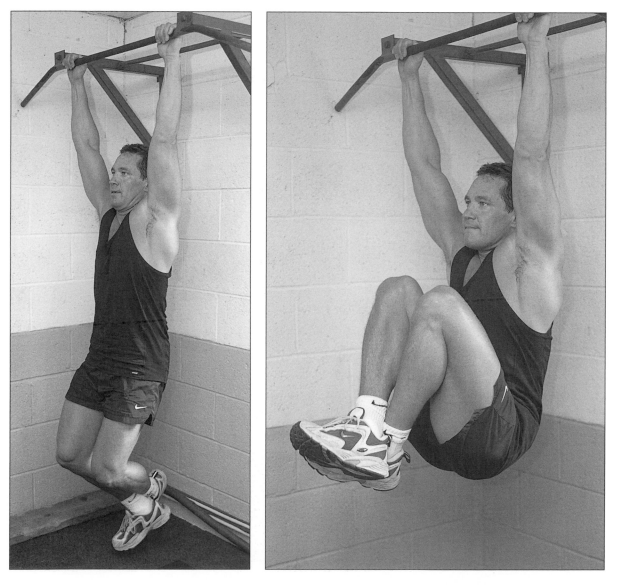

## SIDE BENDS

Stand upright with your feet shoulder-width apart. Bend down and touch your hand to the side of your knee, then switch to the other side, keeping your back as flat as possible throughout.

**FORM GUIDE:** I often use a very light dumb-bell to add a bit of resistance to the exercise, but remember not to use heavy weights because we don't want to build muscle in this area.

**MUSCLES TARGETED:** Oblique abdominal.

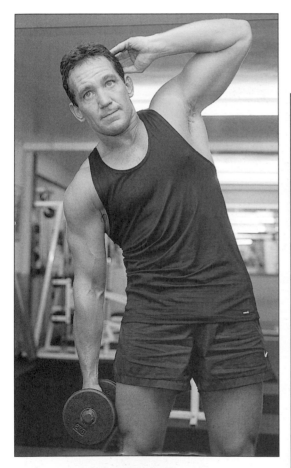

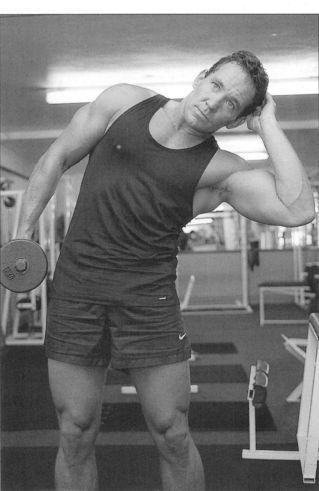

# CABLE CRUNCH

Kneeling on the floor with your bottom on your heels, hold on to a rope attached to a cable pulley. Keep your hands in front of your head and curl your body forward and down until your head and forearms touch the floor. Uncurl and come back to the starting position slowly.

**FORM GUIDE:** You can vary the exercise by curling down to one side then the other.

**MUSCLES TARGETED:** All the abdominals.

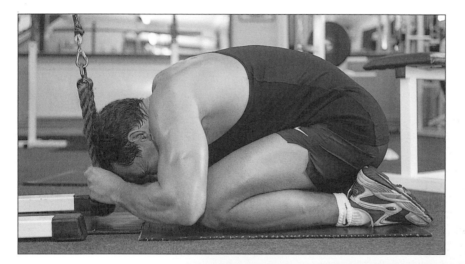

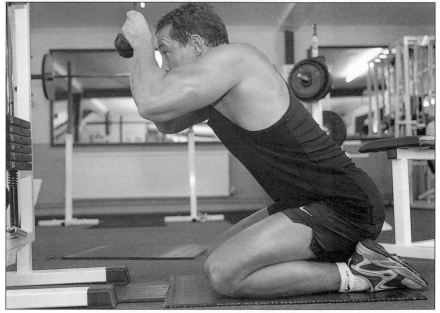

# 12. The work-out routines

## LEVEL ONE: THE START-UP CIRCUIT

This is the basic circuit, largely based on compound exercises which target the major muscle groups and build the foundation of strength you'll need to progress to the other circuits. You'll be working out three times a week – i.e. Monday, Wednesday and Friday, or however you can fit it into your schedule. You'll target all the major muscle groups on each session, working for three sets of 12 repetitions. Between each set you should be taking up to two minutes of rest. Treat this level as your introduction to weightlifting, finding good form and gaining an understanding of how much you can lift.

| | |
|---:|:---|
| **Chest:** | Bench press – 3 sets × 12 reps. |
| **Back:** | Bent-over row – 3 sets × 12 reps. |
| **Shoulders:** | Military press – 3 sets × 12 reps. |
| **Legs:** | Squat – 3 sets × 12 reps. |
| **Calf:** | Calf raises – 3 sets × 12 reps. |
| **Biceps:** | Bar-bell curl – 3 sets × 12 reps. |
| **Triceps:** | Cable push-down – 3 sets × 12 reps. |
| **Abs:** | Sit-ups – 3 sets of maximum (i.e. keep going until you can't do any more). |

## LEVEL TWO: THE SPLIT CIRCUITS

At this level you're still working out three times a week, but the intensity of the exercise has stepped up. You'll begin to target the body parts with more than one exercise and, apart from arms, you'll step up the number of sets to four and bring the amount of repetitions down to 10. With each session you need to concentrate on increasing the weight in small increments, and cut your recovery period between sets down to around 75 seconds.

**EXAMPLE CIRCUIT:**

Monday: Chest, arms & abs.
Wednesday: Legs & abs.
Friday: Back, shoulders & abs.

|  |  |
|---|---|
| Chest: | Bench press – 4 sets × 10 reps. |
|  | Incline bench press – 4 sets × 10 reps. |
|  | Dumb-bell flyes – 4 sets × 10 reps. |
| Arms: | Standing cable curls – 4 sets × 10 reps. |
|  | Incline dumb-bell curls – 4 sets × 10 reps. |
|  | Cable rope push-downs – 4 sets × 10 reps. |
|  | Tricep kickbacks – 4 sets × 10 reps. |
| Legs: | Smith-machine squats – 4 sets × 10 reps. |
|  | Leg extension – 4 sets × 10 reps. |
|  | Lying leg curls – 4 sets × 10 reps. |
| Back: | Wide-grip pull-downs – 4 sets × 10 reps. |
|  | One-arm dumb-bell rows – 4 sets × 10 reps. |
|  | Seated cable rows – 4 sets × 10 reps. |
| Shoulders: | Seated dumb-bell press – 4 sets × 10 reps. |
|  | Lateral raise – 4 sets × 10 reps. |
|  | Bent-over laterals – 4 sets × 10 reps. |
| Abdominals: | Sit-ups – 4 sets of maximum. |
|  | Leg raises – 4 sets of maximum. |

## LEVEL THREE: THE ADVANCED CIRCUIT

This is my personal routine, so you need to be ready to commit yourself to a routine that ties you down to training every four days, the fifth being the rest day (you'll need it!). I use a pyramid system so that as the weight goes up, the repetitions come down. On your last repetition you should be pushing out your maximum weight and, in most cases, you will definitely need a spotter. I try to keep the rest between sets down to 60 seconds. If you find that you're plateauing, then you can swap around the exercises with ones that were detailed in the other circuits.

**EXAMPLE CIRCUIT:**

**Monday:** Chest, biceps & abs.
**Tuesday:** Shoulders & abs.
**Wednesday:** Legs & abs.
**Thursday:** Back, triceps & abs.
**Friday:** Rest day.
**Saturday:** Chest, biceps & abs (the circuit begins again).

**Chest:** Bench press – 5 sets × 12, 10, 8, 6, 4 reps.
Incline press – 5 sets × 10, 8, 6, 4 reps.
Dumb-bell flyes – 4 sets × 10, 8, 6, 6 reps.
Dips – 2 sets of maximum.
Pullovers – 2 sets × 10 reps.

**Biceps:** Bar-bell curls – 4 sets × 10, 8, 6, 6 reps.
Incline dumb-bell curls – 4 sets × 10, 8, 6, 6 reps.
Standing cable reverse grip – 4 sets × 10, 8, 6, 6 reps.

**Legs:** Leg extension – 5 sets × 15, 12, 10, 8, 6 reps.
Squats – 4 sets × 12, 10, 8, 6, 4 reps.
Leg press – 4 sets × 10, 8, 6, 4 reps.
Lying leg curls – 4 sets × 10, 8, 6, 6 reps.
Calf raise – 4 sets × 10 reps.

**Back:** Wide-grip pull-ups – 5 sets × 10 reps.
Bent-over rows – 4 sets × 10, 8, 6, 4 reps.
Seated cable rows – 4 sets × 10, 8, 6, 6 reps.
Cable pull-downs – 4 sets × 10, 8, 6, 4 reps.

Triceps:  Cable push-downs – 4 sets × 12, 10, 8, 6 reps.

Close-grip bench press – 4 sets × 10, 8, 6, 4 reps.

Lying tricep extension – 4 sets × 10, 8, 6, 4 reps.

Tricep kickbacks – 4 sets × 10, 8, 6, 6 reps.

Abs:  Sit-ups – 4 sets of maximum.

Hanging leg raises – 4 sets of maximum.

Side bends – 4 sets of maximum.

Cable crunches – 4 sets of maximum.

'Now follow my lead, get out there and do it!'

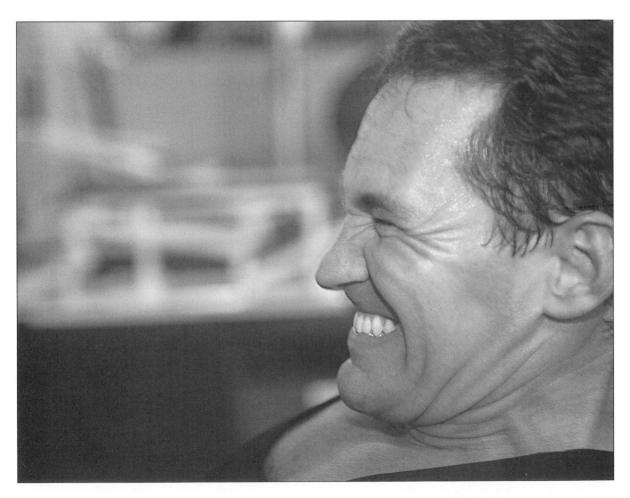

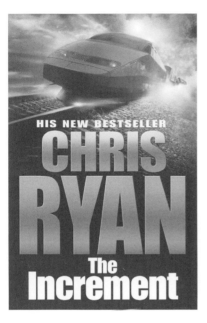

# The Increment

## Chris Ryan

*The Increment – the elite assassination unit of the SAS*

Three years ago Matt Browning was thrown out of the unit for questioning an order – and he was on his way out of the SAS. Now, when he thought he had put military life behind him, he finds himself dragged back into action.

MI6 are demanding he helps a giant drugs company destroy copies of its medicines being produced by Eastern European gangsters. But the mission is not what it seems.

An old friend from the Army has turned into a homicidal maniac – and so are soldiers from around the country.

Suddenly Matt finds himself thrust into the centre of a deadly mystery.

As the answers start to unravel, Matt finds himself the only man in possession of a terrifying secret. Alone and on the run he is up against The Increment – the most ruthless, lethal killing machine on earth.

Century books

*Also available in Arrow*

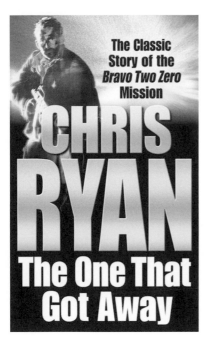

# The One That Got Away

## Chris Ryan

*New edition of the number one bestseller*

The SAS mission conducted behind Iraqi lines is one of the most famous stories of courage and survival in modern warfare. Of the eight members of the SAS regiment who set off, only one escaped capture. This is his story.

This new edition includes an account of the aftermath of this extraordinary story; the way former members of the patrol have fallen out and documentary evidence that settles once and for all what really happened on that fateful mission. Also contains a new section of so far unpublished photographs.

This is the story of courage under fire, of hairbreadth escapes, of the best trained soldiers in the world fighting against adverse conditions, and of one man's courageous refusal to lie down and die.

arrow books

*Also available in Arrow*

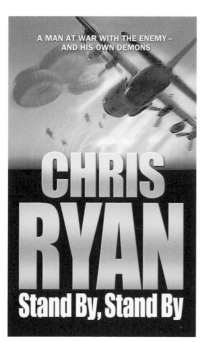

# Stand By, Stand By

## Chris Ryan

*A man at war with the enemy
and his own demons*

The second number one bestseller from the author of *The One That Got Away*

Never has there been a more graphic account of the SAS in action, never a thriller so authentically grounded in the twists and turns of undercover warfare.

Geordie Sharp, a sergeant in the SAS, is struggling to pick up the threads of his army career. Wounded in the Gulf War, he returns to Hereford to find his home life in tatters. As he trains with Northern Ireland Troop, a murder in his family fires him with personal hatred of the IRA. Posted to Belfast, he discovers that his adversary is Declan Farrell, a leading player in the Provisional IRA. Sharp sets out to stalk and kill his man.

arrow books

Also available in Arrow

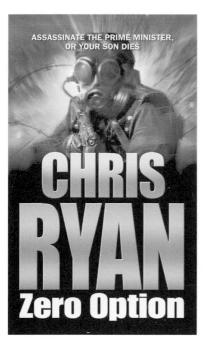

# Zero Option

## Chris Ryan

*The sequel to the bestselling* Stand By, Stand By

SAS Sergeant Geordie Sharp, locked in a desperate private battle with the IRA, is required to undertake two top-secret missions, in the full knowledge that, if they go wrong, the authorities will deny all involvement.

In the first operation he serves as commander of a hit team on a Black or 100 per cent non-attributable task assigned to the SAW, the Regiment's ultra-secret Subversive Action Wing. The target is an Iraqi who defected to Libya after the Gulf War. The aim is to kill him and leave no clue as to the identity or origin of the assassins. The hit team will have to be absolutely clean and if anyone is killed, the body will have to be recovered or vaporised with explosives...

Returning to base, Sharp finds he must also carry out a high-level political assassination in mainland Britain. If he fails, his four-year-old son will die at the hands of the IRA. Trapped between opposing forces in a fight to the death, he twists and turns through a nightmare maze, desperately seeking some way of averting tragedy. Who will be hit hardest – Geordie Sharp or the British government?

arrow books

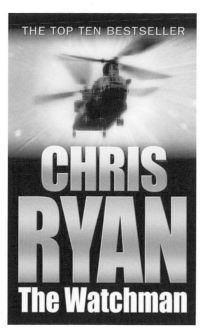

# The Watchman

## Chris Ryan

Alex is a 36 year old SAS Captain. Recently commissioned from the ranks, he is returning from a hostage-rescue mission in Sierra Leone when he finds himself summoned back to the UK. Someone, it seems, has been murdering MI5 officers. And murdering them in a particularly gruesome and horrific way. A hammer is involved, as is a skinning-knife. The security services, however, are more concerned with the why than the how. Because it is beginning to look as if the killer is an insider, SAS-trained, one of the Regiment's own.

The body-count is mounting, and under strict cover of secrecy Alex is ordered to track down and eliminate the killer. To assist him in this task he is assigned an MI5 liaison officer – the attractive but abrasive Tracey Weaver. And so begins a deadly and relentless manhunt. The killer, Alex discovers, was almost certainly an undercover soldier codenamed the Watchman, who in the early '90s infiltrated the highest levels of the IRA's Army Council. He was – and without doubt remains – a lethally skilful operator. But why is the Watchman slaughtering his way through the upper ranks of the security services?

A nightmare chase, a betrayal and a dawn firefight will all ensue before Alex learns the bitter truth: that in the shadowy battlegrounds of the Intelligence wars there is no good and no evil – there are only winners and losers.

arrow books

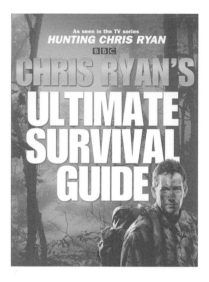

# Chris Ryan's Ultimate Survival Guide

## Chris Ryan

*"Survival means doing what you have to do in order to live, and sometimes that means thinking smart rather than working hard"*

In his new book, Chris Ryan tells us in very real terms what you have to do to survive in the most unforgiving territories on earth. It's not always doing the obvious thing that will pull you through, nor working the hardest. But whatever you need to do, Chris Ryan tells it like it is.

As a soldier in the SAS for ten years, Ryan won renown for his epic escape and evasion across the Iraqi desert during the first Gulf War. A triumph of sheer guts and determination, he pulled through by applying his SAS training to the most extreme survival situation imaginable.

*Chris Ryan's Ultimate Survival Guide* takes us through the importance of mental attitude and emphasises the importance of getting the basics right – right down to the colour of your sleeping bag. Comprehensive enough to be used as a reference book, advice is easy to understand, focused and above all effective.

C